THE DOLPHIN WAY

THE DOLPHIN WAY

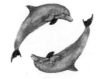

A Parent's Guide to Raising Healthy, Happy, and Motivated Kids—Without Turning into a Tiger

Shimi K. Kang, M.D.

JEREMY P. TARCHER • PENGUIN
a member of Penguin Group (USA)
New York

JEREMY P. TARCHER/PENGUIN
Published by the Penguin Group
Penguin Group (USA) LLC
375 Hudson Street
New York, New York 10014

USA • Canada • UK • Ireland • Australia
New Zealand • India • South Africa • China

penguin.com
A Penguin Random House Company

Most Tarcher/Penguin books are available at special quantity discounts
for bulk purchase for sales promotions, premiums, fund-raising, and educational needs.
Special books or book excerpts also can be created to fit specific needs.
For details, write: Special.Markets@us.penguingroup.com.

ISBN 978-0-399-16604-4

Printed in the United States of America
1 3 5 7 9 10 8 6 4 2

Book design by Lauren Kolm

To Joesh, Jaever, and Gia, my three beloved children,
and to all the miraculous children of this world.
May you journey through life's ever-changing waters
joyfully together as dolphins.

Look deep into nature,
and then you will understand everything better.

ALBERT EINSTEIN

CONTENTS

. . . .

THE DOLPHIN WAY

INTRODUCTION

. . . .

Facing the Tiger in Me

I'm late again. It seems like I'm always late getting to and back from piano lessons, soccer practice, and swimming lessons. My mind is racing with everything I need to do. I've got emails to send, deadlines to meet, and food to pick up. It feels like the list never ends. *I've got to get some caffeine in me!* I think. Maybe I even say it out loud. As my anxiety builds, my nerves become jangled and my head starts to tighten. Both will feel worse after a cup of coffee, but I'm not thinking about that. I'm just thinking about how I need to *not* take the nap that is calling me so sweetly.

I look in the rear-view mirror to change lanes and catch sight of my son in the backseat. He looks so flat, empty, and lost that my heart breaks a little—maybe more than a little.

"What's wrong, sweetie?" I ask.

"Mom," he sighs wearily, barely audible, "I don't wanna go to piano. I just wanna go home and play."

My heart breaks a little more. My son just wants to play and be a kid, which is the way I grew up. It hits me like a thunderbolt: with all the activities, teams, camps, and programs I've scheduled for him, I was turning my six-year-old boy into an overworked, middle-aged man. What was going on with me? Why had I been such a tiger mom lately? You know, that authoritarian brand of parenting made famous by Amy Chua in her memoir, *Battle Hymn of the Tiger Mother*, which proudly excludes play dates, choices, and even bathroom breaks during piano practice. Somehow, I had adopted that same style, even though it runs counter to nearly everything I value and believe in. Then and there in the car, and in a precious moment of clarity, I vowed to make some big changes. I was going to let my son be a kid again instead of some programmed robot. I wanted to be a human again—with vitality and joy, instead of someone running on automatic. So we ditched piano. I confess that I was probably just as thrilled as my son about this new-found freedom.

However, providing my son with the freedom to play wasn't as simple as just blowing off piano. So, where to start? I had always wanted us to play with LEGO together, but neither of us ever had the time. So, I finally took my son to buy some LEGO at a neighborhood toy store. I have such warm memories of playing with LEGO as a child—making houses, animals, and all kinds of wild creations that came out of my imagination. But when we got to the toy store, I didn't find the LEGO of my childhood. Instead, I only found LEGO sets that had specific themes, specialized pieces, detailed instructions, and pictures of how the finished model should look. Children who play with LEGO today know what they're going to create before they even start building. They don't even need to use their imagination! As well, so many of the sets I saw were branded: there were Star Wars LEGO sets, Ninjago LEGO sets, and Chima LEGO sets. Could I find a set of simple, multi-colored building bricks? No.

LEGO started in the 1930s as a company that manufactured wooden toys; it began manufacturing plastic bricks in

1949. Before instructions, LEGO gave children the freedom to build whatever they wanted—spaceships, magical wands, cars, giraffes, or train stations. A few props, such as wheels (in 1961) and people (in 1978), were introduced over the years for children to use if they wished, but LEGO bricks—building blocks for something imaginative—were always the main attraction.

In the early 1990s, LEGO began selling themed sets, which were typically introduced before the winter holiday season, and then often quickly discontinued in the new year. These sets were expensive and short-lived. Where once LEGO sets lasted ten years or even two generations, new themed sets lasted merely one season.

By the mid-1990s, new lines of LEGO were introduced, such as Technic–Tech Play, Technic–Tech Build, and LEGO computer games. LEGO would market and briefly release a new themed set, and parents were expected and became accustomed to rushing out and buying that set at an astronomical price. Parents who didn't get to the store while stock was available or couldn't afford to spend $100 on LEGO every four months were left to feel inadequate. In 2011 alone, ten new themed sets of LEGO were introduced—and were available for a limited time only.

When my son and I got home, he opened the LEGO set he had chosen and we were both stymied on how to put the model together. Quickly frustrated, I sent him off to find his dad. Then we both watched my husband struggle with the instructions as if he were putting together some complex piece of IKEA furniture. LEGO isn't even "play" anymore! Instead of saying that our children are "playing with LEGO," maybe we should say they're "following LEGO instructions" or maybe "watching their parents struggle with LEGO instructions." Sure, children may play with their LEGO Star Wars Spaceship once in a while, when it's not on display, but why not just buy a spaceship that you don't have to spend hours building and can't break in a minute and doesn't cost $100? OK, I'm getting carried away—LEGO in 2013 is a safe activity that resembles play in *some* ways, but still …

The LEGO from my childhood was creative, brain boosting, and totally fun to play with! It made us happy, gave us the freedom to create whatever we wanted, wasn't frustrating, and encouraged us to become leaders who could think for ourselves instead of followers of instructions. What happened? As parents, why do we support this kind of negative evolution? Why did I buy something that was counter to all my core values? Couldn't I just let my son go outside and dig up some worms? I finally realized not only that I could but also that I must, because that's what he really needed.

Lessons My Parents Taught Me

I'm glad I turned the car around that day, leaving piano behind. In the moment it took to make that decision, I was thinking about my patients and my parents almost as much as I was thinking about my son. I had seen the depressed look on my son's face before on the faces of many of my patients— talented young piano players, gymnasts, and math whizzes who were exhausted, fragile, and empty inside. As a parent— the guardian—of a depleted child who was overrun by my own actions, something my parents once said came to mind: "Our children are not our own, they belong to the universe and just pass through our home along their journey, in need of guidance." I finally understood what those words meant— my son was not "my" property, and my job was not to control him but to guide him. And despite all my so-called education and training, I was doing a terrible job guiding him towards what really mattered in life. That thought made me realize how much I value my parents and led me to think about how our lives are so similar and yet so different.

My parents came to Canada from a small village in India—they arrived poor, alone, and with little security of any kind. My mom never attended a proper school, not even grade one; I trained at some of the world's finest institutions. My dad struggled, getting an education by day and driving a taxi by night—a necessity to support his family. I struggle juggling my three young children, my aging parents, my marriage, my home, a full-time career, community service, family, friends, but also a myriad other, often unnecessary, distractions. I hover over my son's grade-one math, while my parents had no involvement in my acceptance to medical school when I was nineteen. It wasn't my parents' instructions that gave me inner motivation, but the values they instilled in me. "Think beyond yourself" led me to speak at local venues to raise money for my own charity fund when I was twenty-one. "Make the world a better place" led me to intern at the World Health Organization in Geneva when I was twenty-two. "Use your creative mind" led me to create an innovative new program for youth with concurrent mental health problems and substance use problems (one of only a few such programs worldwide). "Lead by example" led me to take the position of associate medical director of an emerging biotech company in Boston while working towards being the medical director of Vancouver's Child and Youth Mental Health Programs.

What's truly important in life I learned from my parents. Growing up, I witnessed my parents' profound work ethic—also exhibited by my older siblings—as well as their ability to adapt and innovate, and their unwavering commitment to family and community. Our home wasn't always happy—far from it. Like any family, we had our fair share of stress and discord, including many serious problems. Despite these, as a child, I always felt my family's love for me. I was aware of their high expectations for me to succeed in all realms of life. Most important was their expectation for me to live beyond my personal bubble and contribute positively to the world. The message was clear, and it was woven into the fabric of our home: "Have optimism and joy for life and inspire this in others *so that we can all prosper in a better world.*" This message didn't come from strategy sessions my parents had with each other or from life coaches; there was no time or money for that. It came simply from who they are and what they value as individuals.

My childhood was something parents today would hardly recognize (unless their own was similar). It had no scheduling, tutoring, practice, or even homework supervision. In fact, as the youngest child in a large family, I was often left to my own devices. My mom couldn't help with my homework because she couldn't read. My dad taught me math by taking me with him while he drove his taxi at night; I sat up front, and he showed me how to count change for his passengers. I was in *no* "scheduled" activities—none, not even one, *ever*. I registered myself in school (under the name *Vicky* because I wanted to fit in; my parents found out when they received my report card halfway through the year). I spent most of my time reading books and playing in the dirt or snow. When no other children or toys were around, I played with my imaginary friends. While my parents devoted themselves to putting down roots in a very foreign country, I had *a lot* of free time to feed a growing imagination. I created layers upon layers of stories in my head.

Although carefree, my childhood wasn't without responsibility. Along with my older siblings, I learned to take care of myself, help around the house, buy groceries, budget, and translate bills and documents for my grandparents and other relatives who could speak no English. I was busy—but not in "activities." I was busy in real life. I was expected to do well in school, bond with my family, be there for my friends, contribute to my community, and *always* do the right thing for my fellow human beings. When I was twelve, one Friday I asked my mom whether I could skip helping at the community kitchen on Sunday. My cousin's birthday was on the Saturday, and I had a math test on the Monday, so I thought I should stay home Sunday and study. "I'm sure you'll find a way to do well in everything that is important to you," my mom said. The message was clear. And she was right; I did find a way.

As a child, I had a passion for stories, and I dreamed of being a writer one day. But I believed that pursuing the arts was a luxury out of the reach of "non-privileged" immigrant children. Luckily, I found another passion—namely, the human brain and how it's influenced by social interaction. I became a student first, then a doctor, then a psychiatrist, and finally a teacher of human motivation. But I believe I would have been a lot less likely to have been able to do those things without both the freedom and the responsibility that defined my childhood.

So why was I depriving my children of the simple things— the free time, the responsibility, the real-life experiences that gave me the greatest joy when I was a child and also gave me such advantages when I became an adult?

Twenty-First-Century Parenting and Human Craziness

I've worked with thousands of people dealing with issues such as stress, family conflict, work–life balance, depression, anxiety, addiction, psychosis, and suicidal thoughts. As a result, I've learned to differentiate true mental-health issues from general human craziness. Mental-health issues are serious, common (they affect one in four people), and treatable medical conditions. General human craziness comprises those not-so-smart things we do every day, such as texting while driving, drinking more coffee instead of getting enough sleep, arguing with our spouses (thinking we'll win), and yelling at our children to calm down (and then feeling bad and buying them something). In some ways, these things can be equally distressing and much harder to change. Over my ten-plus years of practice, I've fine-tuned my ability to distinguish when a person needs a CT scan of the brain, a new medication, or a specific talking therapy from when a person just needs some support, more sleep, or to see things from a different angle (or all of the above). What astonishes me is that from all of my interactions with people from various countries and cultures—young children to older adults, homeless people to celebrities—no group displays more human craziness and mindless functioning than twenty-first-century parents. Sometimes I feel like tattooing Samuel Butler's quote "Parents are the last people on earth who ought to have children" on my forehead. Better yet, I could tattoo it on the palm of my hand so I can always see it, since I, too, am one of *them*.

Parents can become afflicted by human craziness for a very good reason. The human brain is the most complex thing in the known universe. With more than one hundred billion interconnected neurons, it processes our every thought, action, and reaction. However, the brain of a human parent is even more complex. The reason? A parent's brain is exquisitely sensitive to every aspect of his or her child's life. Parents are more in tune with their child's voice, smell, facial expressions, body language, and physical touch than any other being. New research in human neuroscience has shown that a mother's brain changes dramatically during her first pregnancy. The amount of neuronal wiring and rewiring is comparable to that which occurs during puberty. A new mother literally has a different brain after delivering a child from the one she had when she saw the positive pregnancy test.[1]

If that's not amazing enough, the father (or adult partner) also experiences similar, albeit less dramatic, brain changes that are triggered by the mother's pheromones (which are hormones the body releases into the air), as well as the newborn's pheromones. Evidence states that similar changes occur in the brains of adoptive parents. For both mother and father (or partner), therefore, parenting literally changes how the brain is wired. It's like puberty all over again, and in my view, it sometimes happens with just as much, if not more, emotional ups and downs. I believe this super-sensitivity to our children is partly why parenting is so hard. Nothing activates the human brain more or puts it into panic mode faster than the fate of our children. If that's not enough, our children's brains are also constantly changing and highly sensitive to our every facial expression, tone of voice, body language, and comment. It's this intricately connected interaction between parents and children that brings life's greatest and most distressing moments.

The Opportunities and Limits of Parenting

I'm fascinated by what science has to tell us about how parenting can positively and negatively affect our children's development. Once I realized my tiger tendencies, I wanted to know: Does tiger parenting work? Also, what does *work* even mean in this context? Does it mean getting my child into Harvard? Does it mean raising a healthy, happy, and motivated child who turns into a healthy, happy, and motivated adult?

Should critical decisions about how to educate and parent the next generation be based on established facts and science, or on individual memoirs about "tiger moms" or any other kind of parent? I had to deepen my own journey not only into neuroscience, behavioral health, and clinical practice but also into my own intuition and deep-rooted values to come to any conclusions about how to parent the next generation.

You would think that, with this knowledge, I would have a clear plan to best raise my own children. Like so many other parents, I often feel conflicted between my intuition and my fear. If I heard that my son's classmate won the regional spelling bee, my fear would urge me to drag my son from digging for worms on a sunny day back inside for some pre-pre-pre SAT prep— despite my intuition telling me not to! I've felt stuck between the proverbial rock and a hard place. Fortunately, my work as a psychiatrist helped me get past my confusion.

Stress and mental illness are on the rise, and young people between the ages of fifteen and twenty-four are the most affected.[2] By 2020, depression is on track to be the number two cause of disease in the Western world, and would be second only to heart disease.[3] Prescription drug abuse is among the top health problems in the developed world, with youth in college being the fastest-growing subgroup.[4] More young people die of suicide than homicide and war combined.[5] Around the world, we're seeing a rise in children suffering from stress, anxiety, sleep deprivation, and insomnia. We're also seeing a rise in children with "overexercise" injuries and concussions from sports, as well as "overstudying" problems such as obesity and even nearsightedness.[6] I know all this because I see it every day, and I know it has to stop. We are literally killing our children.

I've come to believe that the activities of tiger parenting—the overscheduling, overinstructing, overdirecting, overpushing, and overpaving—do *not* represent "overparenting," as tiger parenting has also been called. They represent serious *underparenting*. If parenting means preparing your children for a rich, rewarding life, then tiger parents are doing far too little rather than too much. Tiger parenting doesn't foster a healthy life; I've seen in my own clinic how dangerously unhealthy its effects can be. Tiger parenting doesn't foster happiness; I've seen how unhappy tigers, young and old, can end up. Tiger parenting isn't about learning life's lessons; it's about cramming for the next exam. It ignores the things for which we tend to thank our parents and grandparents and other mentors: the values that will keep our children, our society, and our world strong and prosperous.

I don't mean to accuse any particular parent of getting it wrong. I'm the first to admit my own tigerish behaviors. What I want to emphasize is that there's good news for all of us. Parents don't have to be control freaks with their children or treat their children like fragile royalty. They don't have to choose between a low-achieving happy child or a high-achieving miserable child. I know it's possible for children to be balanced in this very imbalanced world—to be smart *and* happy, competitive *and* principled, practical *and* passionate, skilled *and* grounded, safe *and* independent, persistent *and* innovative, a winner in their field *and* part of their community, ambitious *and* altruistic. Like many parents, I want my children to enjoy music and sports, to have successful, passionate careers—including reaching the very top of their chosen fields if that is where they want to be. Yet, this balance can't be achieved if children are not of healthy mind, body, and spirit. The key ingredients are creativity, critical thinking, strong social skills, positive character, and the ability to adapt and stay balanced in a very unbalanced world. All children should have the opportunity to excel, have a sense of well-being, and be fulfilled with a life that has meaning for them. I think we could see a lot more children grow up into well-balanced adults, depending on how we choose to parent them. Life is not a competition confined to a series of tiger arenas where someone is judging and keeping score. Life is a journey through ever-changing waters—sometimes calm, sometimes rough, and sometimes dangerously turbulent.

Given the state of the world and the tasks of the next generation, our survival on this planet depends on how we parent right now. Only innovators with twenty-first-century thinking can solve our twenty-first-century problems—but they have to be healthy enough and care enough to actually do so. As Albert Einstein said, "The significant problems we face cannot be solved at the same level of thinking we were at when we created them."[7]

Why Read This Book?

I can assure you that, unlike many parenting books, this one won't be adding anything more to your to-do list. In fact, I'll help you eliminate a lot of tasks that you're probably already doing, because parenting can be simple. However, like most activities that seem simple—such as breathing deeply, sleeping soundly, and drinking enough water—parenting isn't easy.

By now, you may be thinking, *Is she really saying that she knows the secret to parenting?* My answer is yes, I know the secret to parenting, and so do you. The secret to parenting is that there is no secret. There is no one way to parent. If you think you've found *the* magical way, wait a few years: your child will change or you'll have another child and need to parent that child in a whole new way.

Just because you already know *how* to parent doesn't mean you're *parenting* that way. For example, most people know *how* to lose weight (eat healthier and exercise more). Simple, right? So why is obesity spreading across the globe? Why is there a billion-dollar weight-loss industry? It's because *simple* doesn't mean *easy*, and *thinking* doesn't mean *doing*. The simplest way to solve a problem is to change whatever we're doing that perpetuates the problem. For example, the simplest way to solve the global economic crisis is to stop borrowing as much. The simplest way to solve environmental problems is to stop polluting. We often know the solutions to many of our problems; the struggle is in implementing the solutions in a consistent way. *Changing* human behavior isn't easy. When asked, most parents would be able to tell you what parenting approaches have worked for their children, themselves, and their families. Most parents have experienced some moments of peace, happiness, and "success" in their parenting and know exactly how those moments came to be. The difficulty isn't knowing *what to do* but acting on *what you know* on a daily basis.

Now, why did you make the choice to pick up this book? That question is similar to something I ask individuals when they first sit down in my office: "Why did you make the choice to be here?" Notice that the question includes the word *choice*. In my office, the responses I've received include "because my parents forced me," "I can't handle all the pressure," and "I just want to be happy." I may say something like "even though your parents forced you, I'm sure you've defied them before." So my question to you, dear reader, is, Why did you make the choice to pick up *this* book? Despite all the other pressures in your life, all the other books on the shelves (or on your tablet), why are you still reading?

I could hazard a guess that you're moving from a place of contemplation (or even precontemplation) about parenting to action. Once a person is in action mode, the rest is easier. How can this book help move you into action mode? The answer is through guidance, not instruction.

In order to achieve our true intentions as parents—to see our children succeed in *all* aspects of life—it's more effective to have a guide than instructions from an expert. And that's how this book is designed—as a guide. I'm not a parenting "expert" and believe there is no such thing because each child and parent is so different. However, I do have a deep understanding of the art and science of human motivation, and I can tell you that the best way to motivate is to guide. I don't sit face to face with my patients; I stand shoulder to shoulder with them. Sometimes I give direction, but I'm most effective when I'm guiding. Nobody likes to be told what to do, especially about personal matters such as how to live your life or raise your children. No one, not an expert—not even a parent—can ever impose motivation from the outside. Motivation must come from within. No matter how "expert" the expert, how startling the research, or how fancy the book, none of it matters if it doesn't appeal to you at a personal level to make you want to change.

The only expert on your life is you. I'll provide insights from the latest scientific research and emerging global trends, as well as stories from people around the world, my patients, and my own life. What you do with this information is entirely up to you. This book is designed not to tell you *what to do*, but to move you to act on what you *want to do*.

This book follows a four-part model of behavioral change— it moves through dilemma, solution, and taking action to reach transformation. Thus, even if you are fully convinced that tiger parenting is not for you and want to jump ahead to the dolphin part of the book, I still encourage you to start at the beginning with Chapter 1 for greater impact. You could skim through Chapter 2, which makes the case against tiger parenting. However, by systematically moving through the stages of dilemma, solution, and taking action, you will be better prepared for transformation by the end of the book.

I start with the basics of a healthy life because neither happiness nor motivation can exist without health. From there, I delve into the three areas of parenting that I believe are greatly undervalued *and* absolutely necessary for success and happiness in the twenty-first century: the world of play and exploration, the importance of community and contribution, and the necessity for self-motivation rather than external motivation (which comes from outside the individual, such as awards and money). I also explore the skills that form the backbone for parenting children towards healthy, happy, and successful lives.

Throughout this book, I offer good old-fashioned "how-to" tips, and even more "how-*not*-to" tips that you can immediately apply to your life. Throughout the book, I use the metaphors of the tiger and the dolphin. Like the tortoise and the hare, sometimes it's helpful to look outside ourselves to be able to see more clearly within. The tiger metaphor has become part of the vocabulary of many parents. I'm hoping to give the dolphin its due. Dolphins have a lot to teach us. They are, after all, known for their intelligence, social nature, joyfulness, and sense of community—the very things I will be exploring in depth.

By tapping into our inner dolphin and shaking off our inner tiger, my hope is to inspire a global community of parents to value a balance between structured activities and unstructured play, between competition and community spirit, and between protection and independence. I also wish to encourage parents who are driving their children from the outside to give children the opportunity to develop their own strong, healthy self-motivation. All of this is actually simple and easy as long as we tame our inner tiger. So, if you've ever looked into your rear-view mirror and known in your heart that your son or daughter would be better off just playing than strapped in and hurried off to yet another lesson, read on. It's not too late to turn the car around.

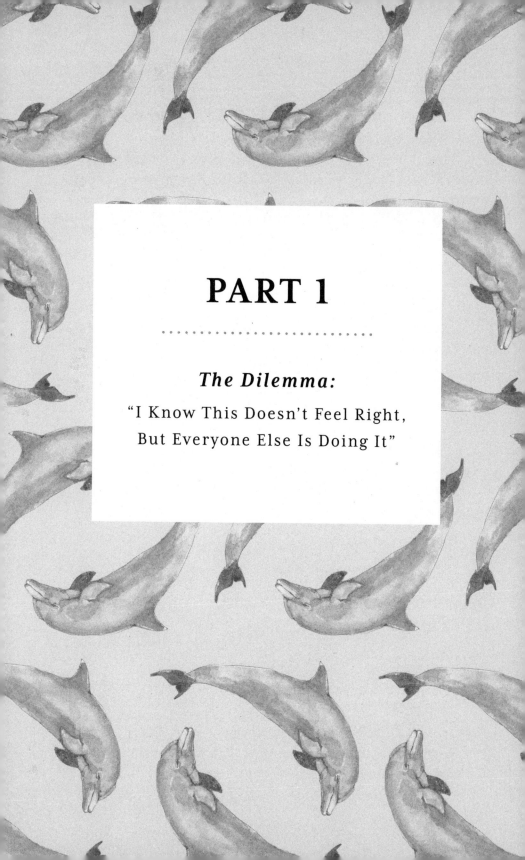

PART 1

. . . .

The Dilemma:

"I Know This Doesn't Feel Right,
But Everyone Else Is Doing It"

Chapter 1

· · · · · · · · · · · ·

THE REIGN OF THE TIGER

In my practice, I have the honor of being invited into the very unique personal lives of the children and families I work with. Sometimes, that invitation doesn't come directly from patients themselves. One morning, my colleague asked me to meet him at an address not far from my house. The police were there. Working with the police is common in a child and youth practice, but this case was unusual. I'd been asked to assess a fourteen-year-old boy named Albert, who had been taken into custody after locking a woman in her own basement. It wasn't any woman. It was his mother. Albert had locked her up for an entire weekend. His mother was safe, and she had had access to food and a bathroom. However, when her husband, who was calling from overseas, couldn't reach his wife or son, he became worried and called the local police. To their surprise, the police found Albert at home sleeping, with junk food and takeout containers strewn all over the house and a pile of video games stacked up by the television. With a strange mixture of shame, entitlement, and defiance, he told the police why he had locked his mother in the basement.

"I just needed a break from her. I was about to explode under the pressure. She's constantly pushing me to do my homework and practice piano. Once that's done, she wants me to do extra piano and extra homework. I know what I did makes no sense, but it was either that or run away or jump off a bridge."

Sounds terrible, doesn't it? And it makes you think that Albert's mother is a ruthless, cold-hearted, tiger mom who is ruining her son's life. Like any story, there are always two sides. This is what Albert's mom, Winnie, told me when I interviewed her:

"Before Albert was even born, I had a lot of pressure to make sure our child would succeed. Albert, like many children, carries the weight of all of our expectations. In China, if you don't get into the right preschool, you don't get into the right middle school, and then you don't get into the right high school, and then you don't get into the right college or university, and then you can't get the right job and you become a nobody. So the pressure began even before pregnancy for me to eat the right foods that would help my child's brain development.

"When Albert was six months old, I was prepping him for preschool admission. By the time he was one, I was quizzing him on body parts, colors, simple counting, and vocabulary. The focus on Albert took over my life. I planned his diet, his activities, his tutoring, and tutored him myself. When I wasn't doing this, I was volunteering at his school or gathering information on how to improve our plans for him. We've now spent nearly all our savings on his tuition plus additional donations to his schools. Because of all this investment, Albert's performance is paramount.

"We *know* it's a lot of pressure, and we don't want him to be sad or stressed. So now we buy him the latest video games, gadgets, candies, and fast foods—whatever he wants to make him happy. But I believe this has led him to become unhealthy—in his body and mind. He has no discipline. He has learned to manipulate my husband, me, and his grandparents simply by throwing a tantrum if he doesn't get what he wants. He has become addicted to video games and now rushes through his homework and practice so he can play. He says it's the only relaxing thing in his life.

"Yes, I understand he locked me downstairs because he needed a break from homework and piano. But I believe he also just wanted to play the latest video game that had been released that weekend. I don't know what to do. He does well in school now because he's only fourteen, but that won't last very long with his attitude.

"He is obviously no longer scared of me, and we can't just keep bribing him to do things. He's losing his motivation. I'm worried about his future—nobody likes people like Albert. I don't even like him. We left China one year ago because we wanted him to have different experiences. Perhaps it's too late. I don't like who he has become or who I have become. I'm really hoping you can help me."

When I tell people the story of Albert and Winnie, they either nod their heads in recognition or shake their heads in judgment. A few of my teenage patients confess that they've fantasized about locking their parents away for a weekend as well! The 2012 case of the American teen who filed (and won) a civil stalking order against her parents (who secretly followed her around her college campus) is just another version of the same story.[1] In addition, plenty of parents have fantasized about escaping from their teenagers—even if it's to their own basement! Chances are, the phenomenon called "tiger parenting" of which Albert and Winnie were victims hasn't left you untouched. Let me be perfectly clear: tiger parenting is *not* limited to a specific ethnic group. Tiger parents lurk everywhere. Amy Chua's book did a lot to associate tiger parenting with East Asian families, but children from all backgrounds are equally likely to be victims of their tiger parents' well-intentioned but ultimately damaging authoritarian regimes. I've seen a number of these children come through my clinic. You may have tried to distance yourself from this aggressive parenting style or felt like you were being pushed into it, based on the misguided belief that it's the only way to "compete."

Over time, Albert and Winnie did just fine. Thankfully, they realized they were both victims of tiger parenting. Winnie hadn't felt right for some time about the way she was raising Albert, but felt stuck because she thought "everyone else was doing it too." Once she stopped looking outside for what to do and turned her attention inward towards what she knew was right for her family, she made better choices. She balanced out the directing and hovering with bonding, role modeling, and guiding, and by doing so helped turn Albert towards a path of true health, happiness, and self-motivation.

New Pressures on Parents in the Twenty-First Century

Like Winnie, parents today confront a perfect storm of converging realities that put undue pressure on both themselves and their children. Some realities have been present since the dawn of parenting and others are new to the twenty-first century. Let's start with some of today's new realities—those that have appeared so suddenly and with such force that we're not quite sure how to deal with them. It's understandable that we all feel pressured into pressuring our children.

School admissions are tougher than ever. Standardized test scores, GPAs, and the quality of extracurricular activities needed for acceptance have steadily risen over the last one hundred years. Today, "ensuring" a good education means involving the whole family in everything from preschool applications to the university admissions cycle. Years before young students even set foot on the campus of their parents' dreams, all kinds of time, money, and other resources have been devoted to the process of getting there. Once the battle for enrollment is won, parents struggle to pay steep tuition fees, manage their own volunteering expectations, and monitor their child's performance, and then hope that it has all been enough to advance their child to the next step. It feels as if one mistake anywhere along this pursuit, like the wrong preschool, could mean the difference between a child's lifelong success and lifelong failure.

Then there's globalization, which is leading to greater competition between youth from developed countries and those from emerging giants such as China and India. Our children are now competing for university and college admission and/or jobs with both our neighbor's children and children from Beijing to Buenos Aires. That means our children are competing against standards of behavior, thought processes, and levels of attainment we may know little about. Will our children be able to compete with the stereotypical all-work-and-no-play memorizers, super-human calculators, and spelling-bee champions coming out of other countries?

Technology continues to open new opportunities and close many others. Major industries, such as automobile manufacturing, agriculture, and even health care, may soon be dominated or administrated by robots. At the same time, our children are growing up with technology, and they're turning to it for information, connection, and comfort. Will technology expand or shrink opportunities for our children as we proceed into the twenty-first century? All that's certain is that technology is here to stay and is ever-changing. And changing us.

With technology comes more connectivity, which, like most things, has its pros and cons. The ability for children and parents to stay connected via cellphones is a great advantage (unless the cellphone is used to stifle a child's independence). In addition, studies have shown that social media can help children who are socially awkward feel connected to others.[2] So it's not all bad. But surely a huge part of our jobs as parents and educators is to help our kids understand and navigate the world as it really is—and even a glance at social media is enough to see that it's far from a realistic lens. Parents don't post pictures of their exhausted selves, their children having tantrums, or their co-parenting disputes. Young people don't post pictures of themselves studying or sharing dinner with their parents. That is, the real, everyday world is tirelessly edited out. What we see instead is the fantasy world in which we appear as we hope others will see us (for example, 40 percent of adolescent Facebook users report seeing pictures of their friends partying on the website[3]).

Obsessing over idealized depictions of other people's lives is exactly what you should do if you want to be unhappy. A 2013 study in Michigan looked into how using Facebook influences happiness and how people rate their personal well-being.[4] The researchers would text message the subjects five times a day over two weeks and have them answer questions to assess how they feel moment to moment and rate their overall satisfaction with their lives. What they found was that people who used Facebook more often had a more negative outlook on both their feelings in the moment and their overall life satisfaction. The more Facebook users were on the site during one time interval, the worse they would feel the next time they were contacted. Direct face-to-face communication between people didn't result in associated negative ratings. Do we really want to spend our time online making ourselves miserable?

Then there's the media. The twenty-four-hour news cycle and the ever-present media are inescapable anxiety producers. We have constant access to breaking news that has nothing to do with our lives. Cases of child abduction dominate the news cycle, not because they're occurring more than they did twenty years ago, but because they keep us glued to our televisions and increase viewer ratings. An even more toxic anxiety seeps into the lives of anyone who compares his or her own day-to-day existence with that of the glamorous and the seemingly "real" people seen in the media. How can we simply be ourselves in a world dominated by sound bites and celebrities?

Advertising colonizes new spaces every day and uses more subtle tactics than ever before to reach us. The average person is exposed to as many as 3,000 advertising messages each day (via radio, television, billboards, the Internet, stores, and product placement in various media).[5] The fundamental purpose of advertising is to make us feel that we need the product being thrust at us. It works by first preying on our fears and insecurities and then offering the product as the means to abate those feelings. We're left with a "more is better" mentality. Advertising and marketing have also contributed to the "expertizing" of parenthood (since when did parents need experts anyway?!). Consider Baby Einstein, for example. Thanks to great marketing and parental hype, Baby Einstein videos became absolute must-haves in the early 2000s. Baby Einstein was touted as boosting a baby's intelligence and even preventing neuron death. However, it turned out that Baby Einstein and other "educational" videos may have done more harm than good. For example, one study showed that infants who watched the videos learned an average of seven words *fewer* a day than those that did not.[6] But these findings haven't stopped millions of parents from spending a lot of money, time, and energy—all of which may be in short supply—to get what they've been convinced is "the best" for their children. We just can't stop being influenced by marketing and experts—can we? Keep in mind that Einstein never watched any videos when he was a child, and he turned out OK.

Family structures and work have also changed considerably. Around 30 percent of US households have parents who are raising their children alone.[7] Single parenting, co-parenting, and parenting without extended family support have become increasingly common, yet our societal structures have not changed in sync to support these families. Work life has also changed dramatically: connection to the workplace is constant, with half of North Americans bringing work home regularly.[8] As parents, we're often so busy with our own agendas that our children become merely bodies we need to get out the door to make it to our meeting on time. For the first time in history, 50 percent of the world is living in urban centers, generally in smaller homes and apartments,[9] where there is less open space. With urbanization comes fear. Paranoid behavior is more common in cities due to the loss of social bonding because neighbors don't know neighbors and children are thus less free to explore. We can't really do anything about any of this—can we?

Then there's the very wide generation gap that exists between us and our children. Is your child better able to use technology than you are? If yes, what does that say about your ability to be an authority in their lives? A generation gap by definition is attributed to "rapid cultural change" between parents and their children. I can think of no greater cultural change in all of human history than what we're currently experiencing in the age of break-speed technology and global connectedness. If Twitter were a country, it would be one of the largest in the world. Many parents would be lost there, unable to fathom the customs or speak the language. Most of our children are even more comfortable navigating our smart phones than we are. Gone are the days of generation gaps marked by musical hits, fashion trends, and political mantras. We're perhaps the most outdated group of parents that has ever existed. So it's impossible to maintain our authority as parents—isn't it?

Perhaps one of the hardest twenty-first-century challenges to navigate is the path to financial security—for ourselves and our children. In the past, the path for one's children was clear. You provided your children with as good an education as you could, which would lead them to a good job that would enable them to be self-sufficient and raise a family of their own. But now, due in large part to the factors mentioned above, we're no longer assured of these outcomes. According to Michael Greenstone, former chief economist at the White House Council of Economic Advisers, "Children are not earning as much as their parents, and I think we're laying the seeds for that to continue into the future."[10] Even the premium placed on higher education may have run its course. Today's young adults are now called "Generation Boomerang." Due to fewer job prospects and longer educational commitments, many end up relying on their parents until their late twenties.[11] And those without a college or university degree are finding it increasingly difficult to get a good job. Now, it's a matter of having the right skills for jobs that will be available in the ever-changing future. But how can you help your child learn the right skills for a job she will seek in twenty years when no one knows what jobs will exist in five years? These uncertainties are unsettling; they unmoor us and make us question some of the basic truths we have lived by. Even the best-intentioned parents among us are confused and frightened.

For all of these reasons, many twenty-first-century parents are functioning in fear mode. We lack the awareness of real choice and become driven by our fears. Think back to the last five parenting decisions you made against your instincts. I'm guessing almost all of those decisions where driven by fear.

Many parents I know have been influenced by one of my favorite books—*Outliers* by Malcolm Gladwell. I can't tell you how often I hear the "10,000" hour rule of practice used to explain tiger behaviors of overscheduling and overpushing in the hopes of creating an "outlier." However, this belief is misguided because Gladwell was discussing 10,000 hours of practice in the context of passion and curiosity-driven learning in real-world settings—not pushed and hovered-over structured activities. The Beatles didn't reach their 10,000 hours in scheduled music class, but from freely jamming, performing on stage, and exploring new ideas. Bill Gates didn't reach 10,000 hours of software programming through private tutors, but from free exploration of computers on his own. Plus, 10,000 hours of practice is only one part of the complex outlier equation that includes factors such as time period and year of birth. Plenty of children have practiced an activity for 10,000 or more hours and didn't "make it." For example, think of the countless athletes who reach 10,000 hours: only a small fraction ever make it to the top.

Recognizing the Tiger's Stripes

Tiger parenting doesn't just take place in a few families with extreme views on parenting. It's a style that encompasses too much pushing, pulling, directing, instructing, scheduling, and monitoring—which a lot of today's parents do! Think about it: How many parents do you know who *don't* hover over, overprotect, or overproblem solve for their child? How many *don't* feel compelled to send their children to this activity and that tutor? Do any of us really know any child who *isn't* too busy?

The sheer number of metaphors (beyond the tiger) used to describe the epidemic of aggressive parenting should be enough to tell us that there's a problem. "Helicopter" parents are always hovering, waiting to swoop down to intercede on behalf of their children. "Lawn mower" or "snowplow" parents are always one step ahead of their children, removing all obstacles to leave a clear path for them. "Bubble wrapper" parents seem to feel that their role is to protect their children from even the slightest disappointments in life. One mother told me she buys two copies of all textbooks so her (six foot tall) boy doesn't have to carry home extra books. How is he going to fare in university, when he has been protected all his life from the horrors of *carrying his own books*?

The three primary parenting styles are *authoritarian, permissive*, and *authoritative*. What many do not realize is that the Amy Chua–style tiger parents, lawn mowers, snowplows, helicopters, and bubble wrappers are *all* authoritarian parents. Whether you are overdirecting or overprotecting, you're underparenting. Parents who follow a mix of directive and protective approaches are definitely authoritarian because they rob their children of a sense of control over their own lives.

Authoritarian parents believe that they "know best." They set the rules and say what goes, no choice and no debate. Xiao Baiyou, also known as the "Wolf Dad," is a prime example of the overdirective parent. Baiyou, author of *Beat Them into Peking University*, became an overnight sensation when his book hit the shelves in China. The self-proclaimed "emperor" of his family, Baiyou writes: "I have more than a thousand rules: specific detailed rules about how to hold your chopsticks and your bowl, how to pick up food, how to hold a cup, how to sleep, how to cover yourself with a quilt. ... If you don't follow the rules, then I must beat you."[12] It sounds extreme—and it is—but the Wolf Dad is not fundamentally different from parents who believe they can prescribe "success" and bully, bribe, or brainwash their children to follow a specific parent-designed path.

Overprotective authoritarian parents are just as controlling because they micromanage their child's every move. The micromanaging that starts when parents hover over their infant to make sure they don't hurt themselves can progress later into interfering with the child's homework assignments, social life, or, eventually, job applications. Please don't get me wrong, overprotective parents are fully dedicated and loving parents. However, by interfering too soon, they don't allow their children to learn from trial and error—an essential learning skill needed to adapt. By interfering too often, they don't allow their children to develop self-motivation—an essential ingredient of independence.

Many of today's best-intentioned parents apply a mix of directive and protective authoritarianism. That may be the case for you, too.

On the other end of the parenting spectrum are permissive parents, who are just as imbalanced as authoritarian parents, but in a different way. I refer to permissive parents as "jellyfish parents" because they have no spine. They commonly avoid confrontation and have few clear rules. Some permissive parents "turn a blind eye" when they ought to be parenting, and some enable behaviors that may be harmful because they want to be their child's "friend." Jellyfish parents fail to define expectations around matters such as respecting authority, social etiquette, or personal values. They may also tend to be the parents who throw open their doors to no-holds-barred teen parties—some go as far as providing the alcohol themselves. Children of jellyfish parents have been shown to be irresponsible and impulsive, have poor relationship skills, and be less likely to respect authority (including teachers, police, and coaches). They often perform poorly in school and in the workplace. They may be more likely to engage in riskier behaviors, such as drug and alcohol use, or get "off track" for a few years (or more).[13] Children of jellyfish parents often float around aimlessly with little direction. In general, when compared with their peers, the sons and daughters (children and adults) of permissive parents may exhibit a lack of self-control, low self-esteem, low competence, and low confidence.

Although what is called "attachment parenting" is not permissive in theory, it can certainly be misinterpreted and lead straight to jellyfish parenting. I wholeheartedly agree with the fundamentals of attachment parenting and the need for a strong emotional bond between parent and child. However, attachment parenting has its clear limitations and drawbacks. With the noble goal of raising a secure and empathic adult, attachment parenting requires parents to be emotionally available and respond to their children's needs promptly. Many believers cite the tremendous amount of "work" for parents (especially mothers) who risk excessive guilt and burnout. In my experience, the strict followers of attachment parenting somehow become the most spineless of jellyfish parents due to their near-obsessive fear of damaging the parent–child bond. Another unfortunate outcome is incredible friction between co-parents when it comes to issues of managing negative emotions and discipline. In the real world, which isn't as responsive to people's emotional needs, these children can become overindulged, entitled, or just "thin-skinned." Worst of all, these parents can often flip-flop emotionally themselves. By trying their best to be responsive at all times, they can feel overwhelmed or under-appreciated, which leads them to behave inconsistently and unpredictably.

Many modern permissive and authoritarian parents (save for those of the Wolf Dad variety, which we can only hope are few) have one thing in common: they overindulge their children. No matter the socioeconomic category we're in, we can't help wanting the "best" for our children. Sadly, the term *best* often means *more*, which often means *overindulgence*. Another term we use for overindulged children is *spoiled*. We may casually say "my children are *so* spoiled" with a humorous eye roll or a laugh. But spoiling children is a terrible idea. When you spoil a movie, you make it pointless to watch. Spoiled milk is not only ruined, it's potentially toxic. Spoiling comes not from giving too much but from giving too little of what's essential. In other words, spoiling is a kind of neglect.

Spoiling children is underparenting. Children who grow up overindulged are more likely to be deficient in daily life skills that require responsibility. They're also more likely to lack important social skills, develop an overblown sense of self-importance, blur interpersonal boundaries, and require constant stimulation and entertainment. Overindulged children have a lower sense of independence, self-reliance, and personal problem-solving capabilities. Conditions such as overeating, overspending, and dysfunctional thinking (such as increased depressive thoughts) are more common among this group of children."[14] Once these same children are young adults, they say to me, "I wish my parents had said no to me more" or "I wish my parents had protected me from my immaturity." Children who are overindulged can grow up not knowing the difference between needs and wants.[15]

For the first time in human history, *high* economic status is a risk factor for youth depression, anxiety, and substance use.[16] I've seen the effects of privilege firsthand. I believe that it's because privileged children often live their lives in a "bubble" that they have trouble adapting to the real world beyond it. High-earning parents may have time-consuming jobs, a busy social life, or both.

The guilt these parents feel about having limited time, energy, and patience for their children may lead them to overcompensate by scheduling endless activities, hiring overhovering help, or being permissive jellyfish who regularly cave in to their children's demands. In addition, children who are born privileged may feel they have little to strive for. After all, where's the motivation to pursue the things you already have? In fact, wealth is increasingly becoming likened to an illness. The symptoms of this malaise are sometimes called "affluenza," which is defined as "a painful, contagious, socially transmitted condition of overload, debt, anxiety and waste resulting from the dogged pursuit of more."[17] The negative effects of privilege may come as a bit of a surprise, but they're consistent with my clinical experience.

In addition, some parents may have "status anxiety," a term coined by British philosopher Alain De Botton that's defined as "the anxieties that result from a focus on how one is perceived by others."[18] It's natural to care about what others think of us; in fact, if no one cared about what others thought, the building blocks of civilization itself (courtesy, sympathy ethics, friendship) would crumble. But worrying *too much* about how we're perceived is a reflection of insecurity. Status anxiety leads us to see identity shaped more by "what you do on the outside" versus "who you are on the inside"—and parents can become authoritarian tigers that overindulge to achieve that image or identity.

Permissive parents hand over control without guidance and before their children are ready. Authoritarian tiger parents take away control from their children. The *locus of control* is a psychological term used to describe where one believes the control center for his or her life lies. A person's locus of control can be internal, external, or somewhere in-between. Children of tiger parents of every stripe grow up with too much external control and thus believe that their locus of control is outside themselves. These children become overdependent on external circumstances and external rewards. That is, they grow up lacking internal control and self-motivation. No parent sets out to rob his or her children of their sense of internal control, which is arguably the key to lifelong happiness and success. Unfortunately, that's precisely what many of us do.

Tiger Cubs: A Lack of Internal Control and Balance

Self-motivation can't exist without internal control. Tiger cubs like Albert (who we met in the Introduction) become increasingly dependent on external rewards to stay "motivated" because they lack internal control. In addition, a balanced life provides the foundation for the self-motivation needed to continue towards new challenges, which is important to lasting success. If one's life is lacking basic balance (for example, lacking sleep, exercise, or social connection), any self-motivation that one has will be directed towards reestablishing balance first and meeting new challenges later. Although an extreme response, Albert locking his mother in the basement was his way of reestablishing balance in rest, sleep, and play in his life.

Ten years ago, in my profession, when we saw a child who was enrolled in an advanced music academy or being given private athletic coaching, that child was someone who was excelling in her natural abilities and talents *and* was happy and balanced. We were thrilled for her and worked with the family to find opportunities for her further enrichment and growth. Today, when we see such a child, the story is completely different. We wonder if he is overscheduled, overinstructed, overcoddled, and overbusy. The push for early overachievement (which seems to be earlier and earlier) has placed children at greater risk for burnout, family stress, insomnia, anxiety, depression, eating disorders, and substance use. Today, in my profession, overperformance is often seen as a "red flag" for potential problems.

Let me introduce you to Sarah. Actually, you already know Sarah. In fact, chances are you know many Sarahs, and perhaps you hope your child will be a Sarah too—at least on the outside. On the outside, Sarah fit the description of every parent's dream child and was on track for "success." Sarah was academically "on top," as bright as they came, and as hard working as she was bright. Sarah's other accomplishments are also familiar points of admiration for parents: she had a spot on her school's highly competitive swim team and was enrolled in advanced placement Spanish. She was highly "driven" by her goal: to get into a top-tier university. But between school, homework, swim practice, and tutoring sessions, Sarah was only sleeping five to six hours a night. All her life, Sarah's grades had rarely strayed below an A-minus, but things were suddenly and rapidly going south. That's when I met Sarah, and once I got to know what was going on inside, I could see that she was by no means on track for "success."

Sarah's parents weren't obvious bubble wrappers, lawn mowers, or helicopters. They were loving and attentive parents who wanted Sarah to follow her own dreams and not their dreams. They thought they were doing all they could to equip Sarah for such a life, to pave the way for her shining future. For Sarah's mother, Lynn, that meant pushing Sarah's talent in sports instead of urging her to take up the traditional piano and math studies her own parents had pushed her into (and which she had hated). By age six, Sarah was involved in a range of intensive sporting activities. Sarah's father, Robert, was focused on providing his daughter with educational opportunities that would lead to career success. The son of small-town, working-class parents, Robert was an entrepreneur whose start-up business had flourished. Nevertheless, he wondered how much better he might have done if he had had access to a better education—like the one Sarah was getting at her school. For both parents, providing Sarah with all of these opportunities was an act of love, and seeing her in so many performance-based activities gave them satisfaction, both in her achievements and in theirs.

Why, then, as Sarah was on the apparent threshold of achieving everything that, in her own words, her "whole life had been about," did she begin to experience insomnia and panic attacks, and suffer from a lack of focus and concentration? Why, then, did she begin using a friend's Adderall (a psychostimulant typically prescribed to treat attention deficit hyperactivity disorder [ADHD]) to help her stay awake to study at night and get through a morning swimming practice?

You don't need to be a doctor to understand that the combination of Sarah's sleep deprivation, fatigue, impaired focus and concentration, use of Adderall, and panic attacks were a recipe for disaster. She was on a direct path for serious health issues. She knew it, too, but there was simply no room in her high-pressure life for rest, sleep, or real help. Getting help would have taken time she just didn't feel she could afford from academics and athletics. No room existed for mistakes if she was going to achieve her "potential"—or so she thought.

After she failed to qualify for a swim meet and took an impulsive overdose of Adderall plus OxyContin (a powerful, highly addictive pain killer she had been given to "push through" a shoulder injury caused by her grueling workout schedule), Sarah became my patient.

Something Sarah said in the first session I held with her and her parents has stayed with me. I think it offers an important glimpse into what it's like to be a tiger cub. I had asked Sarah why she wanted "more than anything," as she herself said, to get into this one university.

"Because," she replied, "my life would make no sense if I didn't."

Sarah was convinced that external circumstances (such as the university she would get into) defined her life and who she was. Her parents were clearly stunned by her words. For a moment, neither spoke. Then her mother addressed her.

"Sarah, darling," she began, "we've never once pushed you to do anything. It's you who decided to focus on all this. This is all something that *you* wanted to do."

"I know you've never said it," she replied, "but everything you do, have done, and especially everything you get happy about has to do with me doing all this #%^$ stuff in a certain way that will get me there. It will make you proud, and it will make you feel that you have been good parents. It will allow you to boast to your friends—which I want for you, by the way, so it's OK. I'm not being an ungrateful teenager, it's just that ever since I was little, my life has been controlled by 'getting to the next level.'"

Sarah went on to say that as a child, the clear message that overrode everything else was that she always had to push herself to be the best she could be. Sarah was sixteen, and she was already burnt out.

Stunned silence hung in the room when Sarah finished speaking. What could anyone say? She hadn't uttered a word that didn't ring true. She wasn't blaming her parents. She was not the product of a dysfunctional home. There was no early childhood trauma, absence of affection, genetic predisposition, or any other traditional risk factor for anxiety and substance use. Yet here was a young woman feeling an incredible amount of pressure to perform to a certain standard, which was not even preparing her for the single goal she had in mind. The harder she pushed, the worse she felt. Sarah was a young, bright, capable, physically fit woman who, despite her parents' best efforts to raise her with confidence and love, somehow missed every message other than this one: your life only makes sense if you perform to exceptional standards.

Sarah is one of far too many young people suffering in similar circumstances. In her case, it took two years of intensive individual and family therapy, plus the occasional use of medications for depression and anxiety, to achieve a complete change in how she lives her life. Now Sarah is focused on balancing physical, mental, social, and spiritual health to maintain stability and her newfound confidence. She will need this balance in the highly charged and competitive atmosphere of university and, more important, in the twenty-first-century world in which she will work, play, and raise her own children.

Parenting without Balance

All humans have a biological drive or intuition to gather, protect, and compete (especially for our children). This drive is all important to our survival—and any parent without it would be a poor mother or father, indeed. If you're not driven to provide for your children, to protect them, or to do whatever you can to help them be the best they can be—just like Sarah's parents— then you're probably not doing your job. However, all intuitions, even the healthiest ones, have limitations. Eating, sleeping, and sex are all instinctive behaviors, and it's not difficult to see how pursuing any of these to excess can lead to problems rather quickly. Parenting, too, is deeply intuitive. Imbalanced parenting intuitions can lead us to a number of tiger behaviors:

- *Overgathering:* Just as some people gather too many things that clutter up their homes, other people gather too many things on their schedule that clutter up their lives. This overgathering is a serious problem for parents everywhere. Our children are way too busy! Just looking at children's weekly wall-to-wall schedules, from baseball practice to chess competitions to debating teams, will exhaust anyone. Children are simply spending too much time in scheduled activities and advanced classes. It's not hard to understand why parents want to give children whatever "edge" they can. However, we forget that humans are also meant to rest, unwind, sleep, take time to eat, and explore and learn through our natural curiosity about the world around us. Depriving children of their ability to respond to these needs means denying them the basics of survival and seriously affecting their motivation. All parents know what it feels like to be sleep deprived. Just think about it: Who's "motivated" for anything when they haven't had enough rest?! Many parents tell me they keep their children busy because, otherwise, they become bored or anxious. These parents are just setting up their children for a lifetime of needing to be busy to deal with boredom and anxiety, which are normal parts of life. Engaging in hobbies and sports is great, but being so busy that little time is left to engage in life is terrible.

- *Overprotecting:* Parents would do almost anything to protect their children, from rushing into a burning building to staring down a grizzly bear to diving into an icy river to save them. However, many find it difficult to let their children take risks. They overprotect their children from life's ups and downs in an attempt to shield them from hardship, mistakes, and failure. Yes, the world can be an unfair and dangerous place at times. However, we forget that exposure to adversity, trial and error, and the real world is precisely what allows children to acquire the life skills that they actually *need to protect themselves* from harm throughout their lives. Children who are overprotected don't develop resilience or self-motivation for real-life problem solving, which of course is what leads to real-life success.

- *Overcompeting:* Little in life feels quite as good as winning, and even more powerful is the emotional rush of watching your child excel. Watching your daughter sprinting towards the finish line shoulder to shoulder with another runner or your son focusing on his next chess move can be almost unbearably intense. But pushing your child to win at all costs, or to see all of life as a competition, isn't helpful to anyone. It's easy to forget that humans are wholly social beings and that we're not always meant to be "number one." We also belong to our community as an equal—in a give-and-take relationship in which we're meant to connect and contribute to one another in a meaningful way. We crave social bonds, community, and a sense of belonging and contribution at least as much as we thirst for victory. Hypercompetitive tiger parents and their children often live lonely, imbalanced lives. Tigers in nature are not social animals; they're solitary predators who are driven to kill with little to no community connections. A solitary life works for tigers in nature, but for humans, a solitary life focused on being number one is simply not enough for a fulfilling and successful life.

Of course, gathering, protecting, and competing are necessary behaviors to some degree: the key word here is *degree*. These behaviors in themselves are not damaging—*overdoing* them is. Why do tiger parents take a natural behavior to such unhealthy extremes? Fear.

When we feel threatened, we intuitively respond by either fighting, freezing, or fleeing. When tiger parents overgather, overprotect, and overcompete, they're simply partaking in modern-day parenting versions of the well-known responses to fear. Overcompetition is, obviously, our intuition to "fight." Overprotecting our children is the equivalent of "freezing" because when we bubble wrap and lawn mow for them, we don't allow them the possibility to respond based on their own judgment, which could mean they'll make a mistake. Overgathering in our schedules makes us too busy and distracted, which is how we "flee" from twenty-first-century parenting pressures rather than face them head on.

Many twenty-first-century parents are functioning in fear mode, disconnected from any intuition other than fight, freeze, or flight. We lack the awareness of real choice and become driven by our fears. Think back to the last five parenting decisions you made against your intuition. How many of those decisions were driven by fear?

The Effects of Living Off Balance

The quick "fix" for fear is control. Performance is something that's easiest for parents to control, so we focus our attentions there. We become desperate to see our children perform, and the earlier they perform, the better we feel. It's like an addiction.

My fellowship in Boston was in the Division of Addiction Psychiatry at Massachusetts General Hospital. Since then, I've gained a deep understanding of what drives, motivates, and rewards behavior, and what leads to addiction. In medicine, we identify addiction by looking for negative consequences, out-of-control behaviors, and cravings. In more than a decade of working directly with addicted youth and their parents, I've seen behaviors in myself and other parents that are similar to addictive behaviors.

Like all addictions, the compulsive need for parental control has a clear cause—the fear created by a deadly combination of the age-old stresses of parenting and unprecedented twenty-first-century pressures. Like all addictions, the desire to control our children is initially attractive. Let's face it—it feels great to have such a "perfect" child. However, most of us, like other addicts, seek control because it diminishes unpleasant feelings, such as fear. Although control can temporarily reduce our fears and we feel good for a while, like all addictions, it takes over. Our intuition, logic, emotions, and common sense can all become hijacked by this cycle of fear and control, and it has brought out a little bit of tiger in many of us—in you and me alike. Many parents move in and out of this addiction (for example, during my first few years as a parent), some have recovered (whew!) but could relapse (my children are not teenagers yet …), and a good number are seriously stuck in it.

I've seen children and parents in the throes of self-imposed stress leading to anxiety, insomnia, substance use, and depression. I've seen young people at what should be the peak of their physical health suffering because they spend every waking minute studying or practicing some activity. I've also seen young bodies harmed by *too much* exercise. One patient had stress fractures in her legs because her parents believed that pressing on through the pain in track and field practice would show the high school coach that she had "the right stuff." Another patient's parents insisted that he keep playing hockey despite two concussions because he was so close to being recruited to the next level.

I've seen young people suffer social isolation from spending too much time on parent-driven tutoring, studying, or practicing. I've seen others who spend plenty of time socializing in highly structured activities (it looks good on the résumé!) with no real social bonds. I once had a seventeen-year-old patient whose entire life was filled with "leadership" activities but who had no real friends. I've worked with children from homes in which the family never sits down to eat dinner together because everyone is too busy, too exhausted to speak with one another, and/or unable to get along. I've treated patients who have achieved their cherished goals—such as acceptance into a dance academy, sports team, or college of "their choice"—but whose lives are utterly devoid of joy. They tell me they feel that they're just going through the motions of life, not really living life. If these aren't negative consequences, I don't know what are.

I've also met with the parents of these children. Almost all of them deny that they are in any way, shape, or form controlling parents. This response isn't surprising; denial is a normal reality of parenting (and addiction). In fact, isn't being in denial a prerequisite of parenting? If anyone really knew what they were getting into in terms of parenting a child (not to mention the pregnancy and delivery), would they still sign up?

Some parents, just like addicts, will admit that they lose control at times. One parent told me how she swore to herself that she would absolutely refrain from talking about grades, flute practice, working harder, or anything else having to do with performance on her daughter's sixteenth birthday. She just couldn't help herself. Others will say that no time is safe anymore. Whether Christmas, Hanukkah, Diwali, or Chinese new year, parents still can't seem to control their expectations of practice, homework, and/or, at the very least, some kind of "planning" for some kind of performance.

Other parents have admitted to me that no matter how well their children do, they're driven by an irresistible—and often irrational—desire for them to do even better (similar to an addict who always wants more). A daughter aces a test and Mom translates that into the need to sign up for advanced study. A son plays fabulous soccer and Dad translates that into the need to hire a private coach to make his son even better. The teacher comments on a daughter's drama talent and parents translate that into the need to submit her video to an acting agency. A son makes valedictorian and before he even writes his speech, his parents are plotting ways for him to top that achievement.

Just like withdrawal in addiction, parents sometimes feel anxious and restless when their children are *not* studying, practicing, performing, or planning their lives; they experience a kind of craving for the child to get back to it. It's like having an excessive appetite; an emptiness that can only be filled by the child doing something we think will advance her performance.

The problem is this: like an addiction, these behaviors lead us and our children to a path of illness and destruction. We can't plan everything for our children's future, and we can't control everything they do. On the contrary, we understand rationally that parenting is a process of loosening the bonds over time and preparing our children for the real world—beyond studying, practice, and drills. In that world, they may make some mistakes and stumble at times, but they will learn to "figure things out" and get back up.

Understanding the rationale for bringing balance to our children's lives and taking actions that bring balance every day are two separate things. Parenting could be said to be a matter of the tension between the two impulses of protecting our children *and* letting them go, and of trying to strike the right balance between the two with every parental decision we make. Guiding us is our love for our children and our insistence, profoundly heartfelt, that we only want the best for them. I believe tiger parents are doing the wrong things for the right reason: because they love their children and want the best for them. It's one of the great ironies I see in my clinic all the time. Parents who try to get their children ahead in life end up setting them back. Parents who try to give their children more end up giving them less. But the tiger parenting promise of nothing but the "best" unfortunately can lead to nothing but the worst.

Chapter 2

WHAT HAPPENS TO CHILDREN RAISED BY TIGERS?

In a hospital emergency room, anything and everything can happen. One night, I was supervising Tom, a medical student intern, and we were asked to see a man brought in by his wife because he was confused and suffering from hallucinations. I asked Tom to take a brief patient history, consider possible causes, and report back to me within forty-five minutes. Ninety minutes later, there was still no sign of Tom, so I had to leave my own patient assessment to track him down. I soon walked in on a disturbing scene: Tom was standing over his patient's bed, and the elderly man was sobbing, red in the face, and extremely uncomfortable. I took over and quickly wrapped up the interview, during which time I learned that the gentleman was in pain from cancer treatment and had asked to be able to walk around. I took Tom aside and asked whether he had noticed that the patient was suffering.

"Well," he said, "I was still going through the depression checklist, and I didn't want to end the interview till I had it all done."

I found Tom's lack of empathy for the patient very disconcerting. I sat down with him after we completed our clinical work to do some teaching. I asked him what he thought of our night together and if he had any questions. Tom completely disregarded the situation with the patient and anxiously began asking me questions about what would be on the end-of-rotation test. In addition, we had seen some other fascinating cases that night—a person with a frontal lobe brain tumor, another with marijuana-induced psychosis, and a high-rolling "sex addict"— but none of those cases seemed to spark his curiosity either. In fact, I concluded that Tom didn't really have curiosity, nor did he have much empathy, creativity, problem-solving skills, or communication skills! When I asked a few colleagues about him, I discovered that my impressions were widely shared by others. Despite many attempts to teach Tom bedside manner, patients and supervisors complained so much that Tom was in danger of failing his internship. Some of my colleagues were puzzled: Tom got into medical school as the highest-ranking undergraduate student in a science program and was a high-level violin player—evidence that he was a hard worker, was disciplined, and had a high IQ. Although others were surprised by this seeming incongruence, I wasn't at all.

Tom is part of a trend I've seen developing among a portion of the medical students I've taught over the past decade, as well as recent graduates in other disciplines. These youth are being called "crispies"—students so burnt out that their self-motivation is charred to a crisp—and "teacups"—"bubble wrapped" students so fragile that they're prone to break the moment they encounter their first obstacle. Crispies and teacups are risk-averse, exhausted, stressed, and rigid—exactly the opposite of what young people should be as they embark on their intellectual journeys. For many whose GPAs, test scores, and achievements in specific extracurricular activities are high, social skills, empathy, coping skills, and creative problem-solving skills are lacking. Common behaviors of this group would include waking up patients or barging in on family meetings so they can meet their own schedules. They're also unable to think on their feet, cope with real-life stress, and solve unanticipated problems. After my own lectures, students have told me, "A lot of youth these days don't care about the concepts; we are just too anxious about what's on the test." While teaching motivational techniques, I've been asked, "Why do we have to learn motivational techniques? We're the doctors—shouldn't our patients just do what we tell them?" (Yeah, right—all we have to do is say "lose weight," "quit smoking," or "exercise more"!)

Although clearly a bright young man, Tom was unable to cope once he was out in the real world of spontaneous action and teamwork. Tom ended up leaving medical school due both to his poor performance and resulting lack of confidence. As you can imagine, leaving medical school caused Tom to go through a difficult period in his life. I very much hope he is healthy, happy, and successful. But with little ability to adapt, I'm worried about him.

The Body and Mind: Reliable Guides
When Life's Off Balance

When I see other children and young adults like Tom, I'm always struck by the lack of balance in their lives. Human biology is amazing. Each of us has a complex and nearly foolproof warning system of biological signals to tell us when we're off balance. But when we ignore the warnings, we court disaster. Biology gives us the feeling of hunger when we're meant to eat, and it gives us the feeling of fatigue when we're meant to sleep. When we forget or dismiss the signals reminding us to do the things we're hardwired to do for our survival, our biology becomes stressed and instead of signals, we get flashing lights and experience discomfort. For example, when we don't eat well, we can become hypoglycemic (having low blood sugar)—and agitated, irritable, and unwell. When we haven't slept enough, we can't focus. If we continue to ignore or dismiss these flashing lights, our stressed biology becomes dysregulated and we increase the risk of conditions such as depression, anxiety, addiction, and diabetes. Our biology speaks directly to us with these reminders, signals, warnings, and dysregulation—telling us when we're off balance in body and mind. However, many of us—including me—don't necessarily listen until we fall over and get hurt.

I was born with hypermobility, which means I'm double-jointed. Flexibility is good, but a body also needs strength—which I had little of. A little early intervention and muscle strengthening would have made all the difference, but neither my parents nor I were aware of this fact. Instead, adolescent hormones led to further weakening of my joints and I dislocated my knees six times, once while just walking. Because of my poor balance, when I was thirty, I fell off my bike and shattered my left elbow, shoulder, and ribs. I had pins, two surgeries, and was left with a torn rotator cuff, bursitis, and chronic pain.

Throughout my thirties, I was supposed to exercise and go to physiotherapy regularly, but I didn't and daily pain in my knees and left shoulder crept into my life. To deal with it, I medicated myself with anti-inflammatories. Eventually, the combination of sitting too much, not enough exercise, and my past problems all culminated into a dramatic chronic pain syndrome that flattened me completely. My right leg had atrophied from underuse, which led my hips to rotate, pulling my lower body to the left. At the same time my left shoulder area further weakened, pulling my upper back and neck right. I was completely off balance, and I couldn't move forward in any aspect of my life (literally and figuratively) until I got the pain under control. It took years of intensive treatments in steroid injections, physiotherapy, acupuncture, and sports medicine sessions to get to the point where I could function again. Once the recovery came, it gave me a new perspective on life. Having been jolted by the despair of chronic pain and disability, I now paid better attention to my health and living a balanced life. In humans, all body parts function independently but are integrated. The body needs balance among all parts, a strong core and alignment, and strength and flexibility. Moreover, it's essential for all of these factors to be optimal during childhood and adolescence, during the prime phases of physical development.

The human mind also needs to have integration, balance, a strong core, strength, and flexibility. Just as the body's most rapid phases of growth are childhood and adolescence, so too are the brain's. In fact, the human brain doesn't complete its "puberty" until around twenty-three for females and twenty-five for males (yes, it's a fact—men mature later). A younger brain needs more sleep and playtime than an older brain. Just like the body, patterns that take root early in the mind are harder to correct later in life.

Let me walk you through Tyler's story, whose off-balance life was affecting his mental well-being. When Tyler was a child, he was anxious. He may have inherited this tendency from his mom, who was obsessed with "what ifs" and "what others think." She hovered around Tyler to make sure he was always in arm's reach, "behaving," and out of danger. Tyler's parents pushed him hard in golf because it was a safe sport, he showed early talent, and it looked good for university admissions. Even though he didn't much like golf, Tyler complied because he felt he had no choice and didn't want to disappoint his parents. Tyler's parents had no idea he was unhappy. The family rarely displayed discomfort outwardly—both parents made a habit of looking "perfect." They also either buried or swiftly solved most of Tyler's problems for him. This approach worked fine for Tyler as a child. However, when adolescence hit, Tyler's cautiousness, lack of problem-solving skills, and internalization of emotion became problematic: he started having panic attacks about different activities in his life, such as writing exams, playing higher-level golf, meeting new people, and public speaking. Each time he had a panic attack, he lost more confidence and became even more anxious, especially in social settings. Tyler never told anyone and began to favor being alone because it felt safer, and found relief in video games and marijuana.

When he was fifteen, Tyler had a panic attack while playing in a major golf tournament. His coach lost his cool and berated Tyler in public. Tyler found the situation too big to solve, so he quit golf altogether. Even the thought of facing his coach or driving by a golf course made Tyler fly into a panic. He felt he had seriously disappointed his parents who had sacrificed a lot and pushed him towards golf, but he didn't know what else to do.

Tyler's panic attacks, anxiety, and isolation became worse, and he smoked more marijuana for relief. All of this led to trouble with his self-motivation, concentration, and memory. Not surprisingly, his grades suffered. At age eighteen, Tyler went off to a college he felt was "not good enough," but still felt unable to get through it. Instead of dealing with the underlying cause of his pain—his anxiety—Tyler self-medicated himself with alcohol in social settings and used more marijuana alone on weekdays. He lost his balance and became seriously unhealthy with regular panic attacks. He could no longer sleep, focus, or concentrate, and Tyler eventually withdrew from all of his family and friends. It wasn't until he was flattened completely with such severe anxiety that he couldn't leave his dorm room that Tyler realized he was in the midst of a major depressive disorder. His depression lasted for almost two years; treatment required significant medication management, individual therapy to improve his personal coping skills and problem solving, family therapy to work though his feelings of guilt and anger with his parents, and group therapy to improve his social confidence. Once recovery came, Tyler had a new perspective on life. Having been jolted by the despair of a clinical depression, he now had a better understanding of how to deal with uncertainty, problem solve, regulate his emotions, and live a balanced lifestyle.

I hope Tyler's example and mine illustrate how our minds work like our bodies, and how both seek balance. Tyler's anxiety was like my hypermobility: because these problems weren't addressed early, major troubles erupted later. I would have benefited from early muscle strengthening, and Tyler would have benefited from early confidence building. The biochemical changes of adolescence set us both off—me with my dislocations, Tyler with his panic attacks. We both went through an event that damaged an already weak frame—for me, a bike accident and for Tyler, the incident with his coach. We both had early signs that we were getting off balance, and we both ignored them. We both self-medicated. We both continued on our paths until our conditions stopped us in our tracks. We both had to put in a tremendous amount of work to regain our balance. Neither one of us deliberately set out to become imbalanced, and it was the opposite of what our parents wanted for us. However, without attention and the needed course corrections, imbalance slowly crept into our lives and set us up for hardships. Imbalance may initially serve children and parents in some way. For example, Tyler's cautiousness helped him avoid hurting himself and made him an easy child who never made a mess. Both of our illnesses occurred because, even though we built on our strengths, we ignored our weaknesses. The earlier in life imbalance settles in, the harder it is to correct. If the imbalance began in childhood, during the body's or mind's phases of development, the body or mind fails to develop in a balanced way, and later the risk of disease, pain, and injury is greater.

Balance—both physical and mental—is something we often take for granted, just like our health. Think of the countless neurons and connections that must be developed in order to walk or ride a bike. In addition, the mind must pay constant attention and calibrate with the body to maintain enough balance to walk or ride a bike. Even though the task of achieving balance seems simple once it's mastered, simple doesn't mean easy. We often don't realize the complexity of calibration until something is missing. The belief that our body and mind will just autocorrect an imbalance is partly true because they are equipped to send us signals when we're losing balance. However, it's up to us to listen to those signals and act on them to regain balance. If we don't, we fall over.

A lack of balance is now plaguing the everyday lives of our children. If our children spend too much time being protected, they won't learn how to protect themselves. If our children spend too much time working at a desk and not enough time living in the real world, they won't learn how to balance work and real life in adulthood. If our children spend too much time studying or practicing and not enough time resting or unwinding, they'll have a hard time being able to relax. If our children are given too much instruction and not enough time to problem solve on their own, they'll have a hard time facing and solving their own problems. Children who grow up imbalanced won't even know what balance feels like.

I think most of us know intuitively that balance is important to the body, but disregard our intuition that the mind needs balance too. Imagine an eight-year-old with an overdeveloped body, such as bulging biceps. Your parental intuition tells you that something isn't right. You may say that those biceps don't look "natural," and you may question whether the weight training involved in building those muscles is good for a child's health. Our parental intuition knows that strength is good, but trying to speed up natural growth and physical development isn't. The same goes for our children's minds. Just as sending an eight-year-old to the weight room is ultimately going to stunt his growth, pushing kids away from natural childhood activities like play in favor of advanced performance is going to slow them down in the long run.

The Obvious Negative Effects of Tiger Parenting
Overgathering Tiger Cubs Are Too Busy for the Basics of Life

A Lack of Sleep, Sunlight, Exercise, and Nutrition Sixteen-year-old Sanjay was juggling high honors, all kinds of volunteer work, and studying for SATs. When he came to see me, he was distraught and ashamed that he had to see a doctor because everyone saw him as being "so strong." I discovered that he was sleeping only five hours a night for the three-month-period before his suicidal thoughts began. Both he and his parents understood the value of sleep, but he simply didn't have enough time in his day to do everything he was trying to do. His parents were loving and worried, but they didn't guide him to reduce his load of activities. Instead, they took turns staying up late with him, made him coffee, and let him fall asleep on his books. They even hired an expensive tutor to help him with his nightly homework when his grades began to drop.

Sanjay didn't need a tutor to get his grades up—he was a brilliant boy. He just needed some sleep. But he was in a vicious cycle that overvalued every opportunity to "get ahead," which only kept him up later, made him lose his ability to think clearly, and led him to fall behind even more. He thought he was going crazy and would end up in a psychiatric hospital, which I agreed could be true, if he didn't get some sleep. He had a hard time believing something so simple, something he had brushed aside for more "important" uses of his time, would solve his problems. When I explained to Sanjay that sleep deprivation is about as bad as chronic smoking for your health, he agreed to simply try sleeping more. Within four days, he noticed a dramatic improvement in his mood, energy, focus, and concentration. Within two weeks, he was back to his normal self and thanked me profusely for saving his life, when all I did was simply recommend more sleep. A recommendation, I might add, that anyone with basic human intuition would be able to prescribe. No medical degree needed here!

At the other end of the spectrum, I've met countless tigers—young and old—who suffer from bedtime anxiety (and resultant insomnia). Because they are so busy, bedtime is the only time their mind has to process the numerous emotions they faced during their day. Ironically, many of these patients tell me that they deal with bedtime anxiety by becoming even busier during their day in the hope of just collapsing from exhaustion when they go to bed.

Some tiger parents keep their children so busy that their children literally never see the light of day. It has been reported that some 90 percent of children in the major East Asian countries—China, South Korea, Japan, Taiwan—are growing up with nearsightedness. Since that compares to rates of 10 to 20 percent among young people of Asian origin in North America, the high incidence of myopia is clearly not a hereditary phenomenon. Researchers suggest that the problem comes from excessive eyestrain due to too much studying and too little time in natural sunlight.[1] Pediatricians are also seeing a reemergence of rickets in the East and the West and believe that the cause is a lack of vitamin D, which is produced from exposure to sunlight. (My guess is that video gaming has a lot to do with it too.) If our children are inside studying or gaming all day, they never have time to be in the great outdoors. Getting too little fresh air and sunshine has serious consequences.

If you're inside all day, you may not move around much, so you're far more likely to gain weight. Childhood obesity has tripled since the 1980s and is showing no sign of slowing down anytime soon. Childhood obesity is an increasing problem in Europe and Eastern countries, and recent studies show a direct link among the number of hours children are in structured, sedentary activities, and obesity.[2]

Diabetes is also on the rise in children. One can only wonder if the increase in "busyness," eating fast food, and eating dinner on the go while driving around to different activities is part of the problem for both diabetes and obesity.

Busyness is also leading to the emergence of extreme, if not bizarre, behaviors. For example, some Chinese students studying for college entrance exams—seen as one of the key game-changing academic events in Chinese education—inject themselves via intravenous (IV) drips with amino acids so they don't have to waste precious study time eating.[3] Proponents—and yes, I'm stunned that people actually admit that they support this kind of craziness—say that the IV drips reduce the time it takes for students to go to the cafeteria and eat, which gives them more time to study. They also believe it will increase the students' stamina and calm them when they're pulling all-nighters. It makes me wonder when the distinction between poor lifestyle choices crosses over to downright abuse of children's bodies and minds. Whatever your opinion, children are getting hurt.

Overcompetitive Tigers Cubs Can't Compete in the Real World

Social Skills and Social-Bonding Deficits Many parents and youth now prefer to pursue individual sports and music rather than participate in team sports, a band, or a committee, mainly because they feel it's easier to "win" on their own. Parents have told me that with swimming, golf, or playing a solo instrument, they can avoid working on a team and have more control over the outcome. A business school hopeful told me that undergrads in her department avoid group projects because they have less control over their marks. Think about it: How many businesses function *without* people working in groups? This shortsighted, narrow focus on immediate performance severely compromises a person's ability to perform in the long term. The world today is just as social as it was in the past—perhaps even more so if we consider our interconnectedness via smart phones and computers. Strong social skills are fast becoming a key résumé item, and tiger cubs lack them. Social skills and social-bonding deficits hurt not only job prospects but also success in every aspect of the word. Humans are social beings, and we need social skills and social bonding for health in the same way we need sleep.

Physical Injuries Children that are pushed too hard and too far in exercise and sports are getting hurt. Emergency room doctors are seeing more and more overuse and sports-related injuries in children. In the 2008–9 school year, 400,000 brain injuries (concussions) occurred in US high school athletics.[4] Concussion rates have more than doubled among students aged eight to nineteen years old participating in sports such as basketball, soccer, and football between 1997 and 2007, even as participation in those sports declined.[5]

The same doctors will also tell you that more and more parents are *not* heeding their medical advice for the injured child to rest and/or take a break from playing sports. These injuries are serious, and so too are the consequences of not allowing injured children to rest enough before heading back onto the rink, court, field, or whatever arena they're being pushed onto. I've seen ballerinas back in the studio despite sprained ankles, tennis players back on the court despite bursitis, rowers back on the water despite back sprain, and skaters back on the ice despite knee pain. But most concerning are the injured hockey players, basketball players, rugby players, football players, skiers, and snowboarders. I see them suffering from insomnia, dizziness, memory loss, attention deficit, anxiety, and depression, all caused by head injuries that aren't being managed properly. When a child is playing a sport too soon after a concussion, more often than not you'll see a parent whose raging inner tiger is making them push the injured child dangerously or stand silent while someone else does. Whether your child "really wants" to return to a sport or you "feel pressure" from the team or coach to have your child back at it before she has healed just doesn't make sense to me. We're the parents here. If we don't look out for our child's health above all else, who will?

Deficits in Character In the pursuit to win at all costs, tiger parenting can lead to children who are overindulgent, self-centered, and unethical.

Cheating and other unethical behaviors are widespread and becoming more commonplace. Children in our most competitive sports are often pressured to do anything to be number one. Young players may "take out" the opposing team's best players even if doing so could cause serious injury. The media provides us with professional athlete cheating scandals almost daily, but I can tell you firsthand, high school and college athletes are often *more* prone to cheating and using banned substances because the more relaxed monitoring practices make it that much easier to get away with cheating. I've often wondered how overbearing sports parents, who hover over their children's every move and morsel of food, could *really* be the last to know. I'm not saying all parents encourage these behaviors, but denial is a powerful thing.

Cheating in sports is just the tip of the iceberg when it comes to unethical behaviors. Not long ago, one hundred Harvard students were accused of cheating on a take-home exam. At the University of Central Florida, more than one hundred students got hold of an advanced copy of the midterm exam and felt no regrets in using it to cheat. Back in 1940, 20 percent of US college students admitted to cheating in high school; by 2010, that figure rose to between 75 and 98 percent.[6]

Recently, I had a conversation with Annie, a teacher of thirty years, which revealed how educators feel they can no longer give low marks to their students let alone discipline them for cheating, especially if their parents are tigers. Annie told me about the parents of one student, Marco, who blamed Annie for catching him cheating on a test and for failing him. She thought discussing the incident with his parents would be a good opportunity for Marco to experience the consequences of his mistake without it being "fatal" (he was in grade nine, and the test score had no bearing on scholarships or university admissions). However, his parents were so worried about their reputation, and the effect the incident might have on their son's transcript, that they launched a complaint to have the whole issue sealed.

Under pressure, the teacher and school agreed to a settlement where the test score remained but was given less weight, so it had no real impact on Marco's grade. More important, all mention of cheating was removed from his file. Marco experienced very little stress from the whole incident; it was his parents that took on the anxiety, stress, and cost of fixing his problem. Even more interesting is that Marco admitted to cheating on the test *and* blamed his teacher "for making such a big deal out of it," which prompted his parents to feel that he had "suffered enough." This example shows how the tiger parenting mentality of winning and protecting at all costs can lead to the breakdown of values such as respect, responsibility, and morality.

Even volunteering has taken on some of the taint of cheating. Many young people simply volunteer to boost their university applications, and will even tell you so. Those who volunteer because it "looks good" don't realize that many admissions officers can see right through that type of inauthentic behavior. Worst of all, those who volunteer because of what they can get out of it miss out on the wonderful feelings of well-being that come from genuinely contributing to one's community.

Substance Use and Addiction In over ten years of practice, I'm seeing more young overachievers using prescription drugs to enhance performance than ever before. A University of Virginia study found that 20 percent of undergraduates admitted to using stimulants such as Adderall and Ritalin non-medically at least once, most commonly to "improve academic performance," "study more efficiently," and "increase wakefulness."[7] Academic reasons were cited as more important than other reasons (such as recreational use at parties or use for weight loss) for using these drugs. In my experience of extensively researching and lecturing on the topic of stimulant drug abuse, dependence, and diversion,

I would say these findings are sadly conservative and the problem is getting worse daily. I see children using prescription drugs to study longer, play rugby harder, run faster in track, lose weight for rowing and ballet, and simply get through their unbelievably pressured and jam-packed days.

Stimulants, of which caffeine is the most common, can certainly improve performance in the short term, but the long-term trade-off is that they can throw entire systems off. For example, the brain's natural sleep cycle can become dysregulated and leave young people unable to sleep, even when they stop taking stimulants. Of course, stimulants are highly addictive and can throw someone's entire life off balance. I've met and worked with far too many brilliant and hardworking tiger cubs that unintentionally became addicted to stimulants after using them for wakefulness, athletic performance, or academic performance.

Mental-Health Problems, Self-Harm, and Suicide College counseling offices are experiencing a growing influx of students who need mental-health services, and there is every indication that the number of students who need such services will increase in the coming decades. Mental health problems such as teen depression have risen five-fold since the early part of the twentieth century. According to one study, an undeniably large increase in mental health problems has occurred among American college students from 1938 to 2007.[8] Compared with college students in the 1930s and 1940s, recent college students score significantly higher on the clinical scales for depression, hypomania (a part of bipolar disorder), paranoia, and psychopathic deviation. A shocking five times as many young people now score above common cutoffs for psychopathology. The study strongly suggests that these results are *not* caused by response bias—that is, it's not just that people are more likely to admit they're depressed today than they were in the past. According to the study authors, the "results best fit a model citing cultural shifts towards extrinsic goals, such as materialism and status, and away from intrinsic goals, such as community, meaning in life, and affiliation."[9]

None of these results come as a surprise to me because I see these problems growing worse every day. Among the most disturbing aspect of these trends, however, is the issue of self-harm. I see too many young people harming themselves by cutting, burning, or self-destruction, including attempted and completed suicide. People who self-harm typically hurt themselves as a way of coping with mental stress. By hurting themselves, they get an initial rush of endorphins, which are released to help ease the pain of their wound. A 2011 study tracked students at eight US universities and found that 15 percent of participants had cut, burned, or otherwise injured themselves. This behavior was most common at the end of the day, when students were supposed to be winding down to sleep.[10]

Suicide is sometimes the ultimate, tragic escape from stress. In the fall of 2012, just before a new academic year, Cornell University installed steel mesh nets on seven bridges on its beautiful east coast campus in upstate New York. The reason? In the 2010 academic year, six students committed suicide, three by jumping off such bridges. David J. Skorton, university president, said the deaths were just "the tip of the iceberg, indicative of a much larger spectrum of mental health challenges faced by many on our campus and on campuses everywhere." Cornell quickly became known as the "suicide school," but it's by no means the only school dealing with this issue. In fact, Cornell's student suicide rate resembles that of other universities and colleges across North America, and it's lower than that of many other schools across the world.[11]

In China, the suicide rate is skyrocketing for college students: it's anywhere from two to four times the rate for youth of the same age who are not attending university.[12] In South Korea, the student council of the Korea Advanced Institute of Science and Technology had the following to say after their fourth classmate in one year committed suicide in the school: "Day after day we are cornered into an unrelenting competition that smothers and suffocates us. We couldn't even spare 30 minutes for our troubled classmates because of all our homework … We no longer have the ability to laugh freely."[13]

In India, if you ask college administrators, they will tell you that student suicide is a serious problem. One study found that in 2006, 5,857 students committed suicide and that this figure increased by 26 percent in 2010 to 7,379 (or roughly twenty students a day).[14]

Of course, suicide is an extremely complex issue that rarely has a single trigger. In fact, all mental health issues among young people are the result of an interaction of multiple factors such as genetics, early childhood experiences, trauma, head injuries, personality, hormones, substance use, and environment. So, I'm not saying that we should blame tiger parenting for all of young people's unhappiness. In fact, it would be more accurate to say that the imbalanced "tiger culture" many of us live in now factors the most into unhappiness.

Most disheartening is that some of our brightest and most talented youth are at highest risk for self-harm and suicide. Children who excel early in academics, sports, or music are plucked out and smothered with classes, tutors, and incredible expectations to perform, often at all costs. Their sense of self increasingly depends upon achievement. Their locus of control becomes fully and squarely external. Many of these "high achievers" see any form of failure—in a test, a competition, or a

friendship—as a catastrophe, not as the valuable learning experience it can be. They have no clue how to cope with failure, which
is a natural part of life, because they have never been allowed to
fail. In addition, many have told me that their parents and others
may turn a blind eye to self-destructive behaviors. They say "as
long as I ... [fill in the blank: get good grades, make the football
team, win medals for piano, etc. ...], I can pretty much do what
I want." Unfortunately, no one wants to rock the boat of a future
star, even if that boat is slowly sinking.

As a psychiatrist, I've experienced the devastation of suicide
too often and too closely. These stories and statistics really are
just the tip of the iceberg. Regardless of how high or low the
numbers get, even the loss of one more bright young mind is
more than the world can bear. The entire world mourns along-
side the parents of these children who senselessly left us before
their time.

How Tiger Parenting Backfires

The cumulative day-to-day and long-term effects of tiger
parenting move children away from the success their parents want
for them. I'm referring not only to career achievement but also
to physical, mental, social, and spiritual health and well-being.

Su Yeong Kim, an associate professor of human development and family sciences at the University of Texas, followed
more than 300 Chinese American families for eight years.[15] She
looked at why tiger parenting may work for Chinese American
families when that same harsh parenting style was proven to be
damaging to non-Asian children.

As it turns out, tiger parenting doesn't work for anyone. Kim
discovered that most Chinese American parents aren't really the

authoritarian tigers one might expect after reading *Battle Hymn of the Tiger Mother*.[16] And, more important, harsh, emotionally disengaged Chinese American parents end up with children who are just as miserable and rudderless as the children of tiger parents of other ethnicities. The children of parents whom Kim classified as "tiger parents" had lower academic achievement and educational attainment, as well as greater psychological maladjustment and family alienation than the children of parents characterized as "supportive" or "easygoing." The children of supportive parents had the best developmental outcomes, as measured by academic achievement, educational attainment, and family integration. These children also avoided the academic pressure, depressive symptoms, and parent–child alienation suffered by their tiger peers. Kim's study leaves no doubt that tiger parenting comes with huge costs and little payoff.

Tiger Cubs Aren't Ready for the Twenty-First-Century World

The basic structure and methodology of schooling has changed little since the early nineteenth century, when the Kingdom of Prussia introduced the first compulsory state-funded school system. Its emphasis was on obedience, duty, and military readiness—and it worked so well that it quickly spread across Europe and North America, where it remains the foundation of today's schools. Not surprisingly, our children are being thoroughly prepared for the intellectual challenges of the previous two centuries.

During the nineteenth century and most of the twentieth, information was nowhere near as accessible as it is now, and people with the most knowledge were the most valued. Test scores and grades were an easy way to identify those with the most knowledge. Thus, schools began to focus on test scores and so too did parents, who often pushed their children to get the best possible marks. And a hundred years ago, that made perfect sense.

Today, technology and machines, the same things that spawned the traditional classroom and equated intelligence with high test scores, have made that classroom style outdated. Because of technology, it's no longer about knowing the right answer, it's about *asking* the right questions. The nineteenth-century educational model turned children into machines. (In fact, the word *computer* was originally applied to humans who performed complex mathematical calculations before the arrival of the electronic calculator. In the nineteenth century, teams of bright young men and, by World War II, women, would sit down with pencil and paper to crunch the numbers now churned out by computers.) Along the way, the machine became the model human: "she's a *machine*" is an expression of praise. The trouble is, humans are not machines, and we're no longer better at being machines than machines are. Machines can spell faster, calculate faster, and find information faster than we can. What children need to succeed in the twenty-first century are cognitive skills that computers don't have: imagination and creativity, as well as the ability to collaborate, think critically, communicate, and innovate.

We don't need to know all the data, but we do need to be able to tell the good data from the bad. We don't need the answer to every question, but we do need to know where to find the right answer in the dense thicket of wrong answers. We can't be expected to figure everything out on our own, but we can certainly be expected to draw on someone else's work without stealing it. Collaboration, interpretation, and ethics—these are the things machines don't do, but our children should.

It's becoming increasingly obvious that technology may be forcing us to think wider and broader than ever before. Fifteen years ago, Google, Facebook, and Twitter didn't exist. Now, can you imagine your world without them? Who knows which companies that don't exist today will be so essential that in ten years their names will be added to the dictionary (or, should I say, Dictionary.com!). Just five years ago, social media managers, user experience (UX) designers, and cyborg anthropologists were unheard of. Consider the fact that a child starting grade one in 2014 will graduate from university in around 2029. How can we possibly prepare our children to work in twenty-first-century fields that haven't yet been developed using twenty-first-century technologies that are just being dreamed of if we keep on teaching them nineteenth-century skills? That's exactly what's happening. We're giving them the tools they *don't* need to succeed.

At this point, you might say, "the system may be outdated, but that's the system my kids are in, so they're going to have to live with it." Well, thankfully things are changing. University deans are wringing their hands, wondering what to do with the current crop of incoming crispies and teacups, and they realize that the admissions process is deeply flawed—because it often rewards those who are nineteenth-century test-takers, not twenty-first-century thinkers.

A 2011 report from the University of Southern California and the Education Conservancy makes a compelling argument for refocusing the admissions process.[17] The report comes down pretty hard on the current college and university admissions processes, which, the authors write, "bestows unwarranted value to standardized tests as a supreme measure of academic competence, creating the impression that test scores are more important than a student's actual learning or development, and giving rise to multi-billion dollar industries in testing, test-prep, and test coaching."[18] In addition, the authors state that the admissions process "reinforces a cynical attitude in students that gaining admission to a selective institution is an end in itself rather than the beginning of an educational journey—an attitude that gives rise to widespread cheating and gaming the system in high school while contributing to a weakened demand for effective teaching and a devaluation of learning in college."[19] They also call for a new test template for evaluating high school students' readiness for college based on their personal desire to learn and excel in higher education.

We're only at the beginning of what will hopefully be a seismic shift. Ironically, one of the strong motivators for tiger parents is obtaining job security for their children, and that's the area in which tiger parenting may be backfiring the most.

Tiger Cubs Underperform in the Twenty-First-Century Workplace

The great promise of tiger parenting is that it's the right approach for an increasingly competitive world. It's true that the work world our children will enter will be far different from ours, but not in the way the tiger parenting model expects. The twenty-first century is globally competitive and technologically connected, but it's also increasingly social. Moreover, when surveyed, more than 1,500 of the world's leading chief executive officers identified creativity as the most important leadership characteristic for the twenty-first century[20]—a characteristic that tiger parenting stifles.

Employers are complaining that new young hires or young graduates can't think creatively, work through a problem, or work together. The well-rounded individuals advertised in polished résumés don't necessarily exist in the flesh. This incongruence is due to the fact that the definition of *well-rounded* has been misinterpreted by tiger parents. "Well-rounded" has become less about a person's exploration of different areas based on their natural interests and more about a parent-driven requirement. A tiger cub's exploration of an activity is *instruction* in that activity. For tiger cubs who will be applying to high school, college, or graduate school, being "well-rounded" means undertaking yet another adult-instructed résumé-building activity.

Diverse experiences—from music to team sports—help develop qualities such as diligence, creativity, and quick thinking, all of which lead to greater productivity and innovation. But if the motivation to participate in such experiences is externally driven, the positive qualities associated with them don't develop. By the time students are in college or graduate school, it's far too late to try to develop those qualities.

Unhappy, on edge, anxious, and unprepared for the real world, today's youth (the cohort born after 1980) have become known as "Generation Entitled" and "Gen Y"—as in "Y can't I have what I want?" You might be thinking that people have been shaking their heads over the shortcomings of each contemporary generation since the beginning of human history. "Children these days" have always driven their elders crazy. But this time, the elders just may be right. Recent studies have found that Generation Y is quantifiably different from previous generations. Generation Y has been shown to rank values such as community involvement and self-acceptance much lower than wealth attainment, personal image, and fame. These young people— also sometimes called *Millennials*, *Gen Me*, or *Gen Entitled*— are less willing to donate to charity, protect the environment, or get involved in social causes. On the upside, the Millennials are also more extroverted (although that doesn't necessarily mean they have better social skills), less sexist, and less prejudiced than previous generations (except when it comes to people who are overweight). Interestingly, that lack of prejudice has less to do with empathy and more to do with tolerance.[21]

Generation Y's strong sense of entitlement is causing real problems in the workplace. Employers now routinely complain that Gen Y workers are cocky, believe the rules don't apply to them, and don't feel it's necessary for them to "pay their dues." Companies such as Merrill Lynch and Ernst & Young are actually hiring consultants to help them train their Millennial workers.[22] Those consultants may have their work cut out for them. One study showed that this cohort would rather be unemployed than accept a job they think is beneath them, and that on average they considered thirty to be the right age to move out of their parents' homes (no doubt the two facts are related).[23]

Business leaders and human resources managers everywhere are frustrated with young employees who can't "think outside the box," find solutions to problems, or (even worse) have their parents negotiate their contracts or call in sick for them. Managers note that many young employees are poor collaborators because they're too competitive or lack important social skills, or both. A chief executive officer of a top corporation told me, "Many applicants have perfect lives, and many have even achieved high levels in academics, music, and sports. But it only counts if they can also collaborate and innovate. In fact, it actually may count *against* them—as an indication that they lived in some kind of bubble with no real-life experience. If I get that feeling from an applicant, I just cross that person out." Twenty-first-century employers can now see tigers from miles away—literally.

The Personal Cost of Being a Tiger Parent

Those of us who've been caught up in the tiger culture have had the best intentions, but we simply haven't done well enough for our children. And what about for ourselves? Are we benefiting from the tiger lifestyle? Far from it!

In my case, tiger parenting almost cost me my precious daughter. My husband and I had two healthy children when the "third child" question started to rage in my mind. Even though our lives were already out of control with all the schedules, hovering, and cost of two children, something inside me wanted another child. My husband (the practical one) was clear: "No, our lives are already too hectic and too costly. We simply can't afford another child. We will go crazy, broke, or both." Intellectually, I agreed with him. There was just no room for another child in our lives. That's when it clicked for me: our lives had become completely off balance. As I said to my husband, "If my parents could raise five children successfully with far less, I'm sure we can raise three. I'm not exactly sure how we'll do it, but I know we can." To do so, of course, we needed to tame the tiger inside of us.

My mom always told me that if I wanted something purely and with a clean heart, not for any other external reason, I would find a way to get it. I wanted a third child purely and with a clean heart, and not for any external reason. In fact, I knew a third child would be a big blow to all the external things I valued so much: my career (after two maternity leaves, the program I had created was unravelling), my appearance (I hadn't lost the extra pounds from my last pregnancy yet and I had pretty much looked exhausted for the past four years), my financial status (Who can afford three children these days?), my house (it would become an even bigger mess), my social status (we would be one of those overwhelmed three-children families that no one invites over), and even some of my friendships. Plus, another pregnancy certainly wouldn't help my marriage, my bad knees, my bad back, and my need for sleep!

I guess it's only when you want something so wholly that you're willing to look honestly and deeply into what's standing in the way of getting it. Once I did, I realized the main thing standing in the way of having a third child was me and the unsustainable life I had created for myself and my family. Of course, my husband was in on it too. In fact, control was even more important to him than me (his dad's side was in the military). But I'm the Medical Director of Child and Youth Mental Health for a whole city, and I'm the expert in self-motivation, not him. I should have known better than to do the very things that weren't just pointless, but harmful to my family.

After the birth of my first child, as a nervous new mom, I started tiger parenting out of fear. Then I just continued out of mindlessness and convenience. Although it's physically and financially depleting, tiger parenting requires little emotional work. Tiger parents are so caught up in the busyness of their lives that they stay at arm's length from their children. Tiger parenting lets us sidestep deep emotions such as vulnerability, compassion, and unconditional acceptance. Tiger parents work hard, but they don't work smart. If they did, they would pay closer attention to the things that really matter and understand that not noticing those things costs both parents and children alike.

I finally looked inward and admitted to myself and to my husband that we were living imbalanced tiger lives. In response, we decided to change our lives and regain our balance. It wasn't easy, and it was definitely scary at times. But life is a journey through ever-changing waters, not a series of competitions. We're now swimming in those waters, sometimes peacefully, sometimes playfully, sometimes cautiously, and many times with difficulty. But we're doing it together, with our three children (my wonderful baby girl included).

Tiger families undergo a lot of pain raising children. To start with, all those lessons and all that tutoring cost a lot of money, and paying for these expenses can cause a lot of stress. What's more, time spent driving a child here, there, and everywhere—to swim meets or music lessons or tutoring—is time taken away from income-earning activities, household chores that pile up, other children who may feel left out, other relationships, marriage, family, "me" time, and, most important, quality time with your child. A tiger family may have a father–son duo involved in one activity and a mother–daughter duo involved in another. As a result, family members live parallel lives, and the house becomes a pitstop versus an actual nurturing home. In addition, tiger parents often burn out, typically during their child's teenage years, a particularly important time for them to be present. With this kind of lifestyle, children, parents, and especially the family unit all suffer. I've experienced this suffering myself and seen it in others too many times. By all accounts—my own observations and those of my colleagues in health, education, science, and research, and especially those of parents and children—the problem is just getting worse and it must, and can, be stopped.

Taming the Tiger Within

If the tiger-parenting model isn't working, and if it's scarring our children (and parents too) in ways seen and unseen, how can we prepare our children to succeed in the twenty-first century? Is there a better model, one that will increase children's chances of being healthy, happy, self-motivated, and truly successful leaders that will contribute to the world?

Yes, there is! But before I tell you what this model is, I must first ask you some hard questions so you can prepare yourself to tame your tiger or the tigers around you. Here is your self-exam:

- *What are your real expectations of your children?* You probably have high expectations for them to get a good job and make a good living. But do you have expectations for their happiness? For their ability to innovate or use their creativity? For their ethics and sense of community? If your expectations are only about performance or short-term success, you're asking them to settle for what looks like immediate gains while sacrificing the chance for the kind of sustainable achievements that can enrich and enhance life over the long term.

- *Do you feel the need to keep up with the Joneses, the Chans, the Guptas, or the Kardashians (almost all of us do, so don't feel ashamed of admitting it)?* To some degree, we've accepted that outside tokens—our house, our car, and our children's appearance and performance— are standards by which we measure ourselves. For some families, a child in an Ivy League school is like a Ferrari in the driveway or a Louis Vuitton bag on the shoulder. It says something about *you*—about your success, your discernment, your superb taste, and your ability to afford the tuition fees. Keeping up is about the fear of missing out or being left out. It puts us in flight mode and we overgather and become too busy in response.

- *Do you want to be perfect?* It's hard not to, given the way the media—and social media—showcase perfection as ideal and desirable. The problem is, of course, that the idea we can achieve perfection is a distortion of reality. Perfection is a myth and a huge obstacle for real success. Perfectionists typically have a fear of failure, which prevents them from solving problems with trial and error, and leads them to avoid taking risks and especially displaying the sort of vulnerability that makes people "real."

- *Are your children overscheduled?* It's great for children to pursue a range of activities, but how many is too many—or how much time spent at activities is too much time? Shouldn't there be room for free time—for children to relax, to be by themselves for a bit to ponder this or that, even to become bored? Children today have *half* the free time they did thirty years ago.[24] Many parents tell me, "but my children *want* to be in all these activities—they're *begging me* to sign them up!" That's because for many of them who started their busy schedule at age two or three, activities are all they know. They don't know how to handle rest or cope with boredom, and they have little imagination for finding ways to relax, have fun, or learn on their own.

- *Are your children's lives overstructured?* Seeing to it that your children have the tutoring or coaching they need is great, but not if it takes over the learning process and intrudes into time for exploration they would do on their own. A life that's too structured is stifling, and being instructed in everything leaves no room for creativity and the ability to think through a problem and solve it.

- *Are you pushing your children too hard?* Of course, everybody needs a tailwind of encouragement. However, pushing children too much impedes the development of their self-motivation. They can end up resenting the mandate you've created for them; worse, they may fail to develop a sense of who they are and self-motivation.

- *Are you hovering?* All children need to be watched, protected, helped, and rescued from time to time. Are you encouraging the process of independence *from* you or *towards* you? Are you taking over tasks that your children need to learn, whether it be picking out your children's clothes, classes, or careers?

- *Are you paving the way for your children without letting them share the job?* Sure, it's great to lay the foundation that can enable your children to rise to the occasion. Do you step in too soon and/or too often? If so, you may be depriving your children of the chance to deal with adversity, experience natural consequences, figure things out on their own, and learn from being challenged.

Maybe you do none of these things and still feel that something is not quite right. In that case, perhaps it's not you that's the tiger. Children can do these things to *themselves*. It's in the air and part of the culture. The fear of wasting time, the pursuit of perfectionism, the desire to keep up with others, and the expectations to get high grades and make good money are everywhere. The result is that many young people mindlessly pursue externally driven goals of individual performance at the expense of internal goals of mental, physical, and social health—without any prodding from their parents. A young patient once told me, "I am my own tiger mom."

Wherever it shows up, tiger culture isn't sustainable, and it's not good for children, parents, or society at large. While we owe it to our children to maximize every opportunity available to them, parenting doesn't mean battling against the realities of the world around us. It means *navigating* them. To do so, we must be calm, attentive, strong, and adaptive. If you want your child to grow up to be healthy, happy, and self-motivated (and what parent doesn't?), you'll have to shake off the tiger and embrace the dolphin.

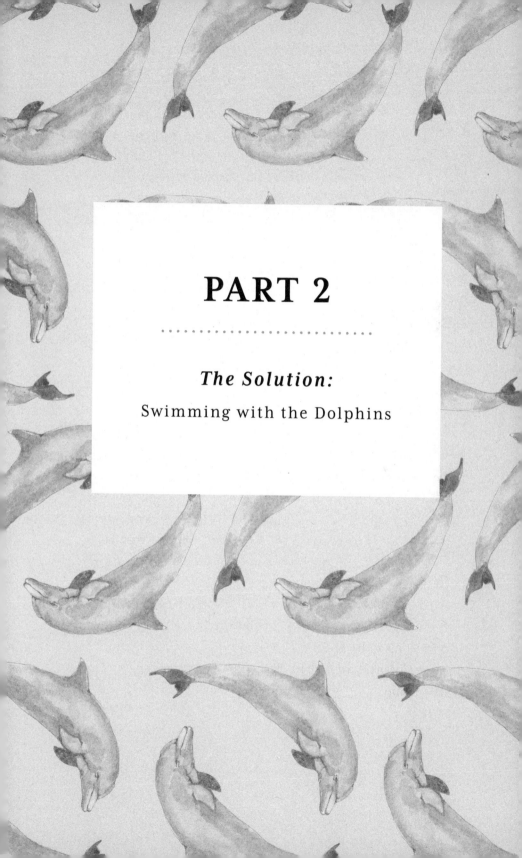

PART 2

· ·

The Solution:

Swimming with the Dolphins

Chapter 3

THE TWENTY-FIRST CENTURY
IS THE AGE OF THE DOLPHINS

South Korea has been at war with North Korea for over fifty years. Across the width of the Korean peninsula, South Korean soldiers have been locked in a battle of wills with one of the biggest armies in the world, led by what is possibly the planet's most unpredictable regime. Illegal nuclear tests, naval incursions, and unprovoked artillery attacks are regular features of life in South Korea. Seoul, the sprawling modern metropolis of nearly ten million people, is within range of North Korean artillery. The South–North Highway is studded with defensive fortifications. South Korea's armed forces are kept on high alert, and for good reason. The country faces the threat of apocalyptic war every day.

Naturally, South Koreans take military defense very seriously, from their missile defense systems and next-generation fighters to their modern navy. And none of this is cheap. At about 2.8 percent of GDP, the South Korean defense budget in 2012 was proportionally bigger than China's or that of NATO powers like the United Kingdom, France, or Germany.[1] That's a lot of money, but then you would expect a country to spend its resources on things they deem most important. And avoiding annihilation seems like a wise priority.

If you can tell what a nation's priorities are by its spending, it becomes pretty clear how South Koreans feel about school— specifically, getting into a particular school. If students aren't accepted into the "right" institution (preschool or anything above), they'll often embark on intense and grueling tutoring (up to fourteen hours a day) for an entire year to try to retake the tests and gain admission the next year.[2] In 2010, 74 percent of all South Korean students were involved in some sort of after-school tutoring. Students are known to take all-night classes and also have their beds removed by their parents to prevent sleeping instead of studying. The exhaustion, stress, anxiety, depression, substance use, and suicide problems became so bad that in 2010 the government had to step in and pass a curfew in 2010, mandating tutoring institutions in Seoul to close at 10 P.M. in hopes that the tortured students would be sent home (even if there was no bed for them to sleep in).[3] Even so, kids' lives are still spent in a bleary-eyed whirl between school and tutors. So huge and entrenched is the country's investment in supplementary education that a staggering 2 percent of South Korea's GDP is spent on tutoring alone![4]—nearly as much as the country spends on its standoff with its nuclear-armed enemy to the north.

It's natural to ask, Is it all worth it? All that time and money, all those precious weekends and sunny afternoons of childhood spent hunched over a desk rather than at play outside. South Koreans sacrifice a great deal to accomplish something they clearly feel is crucial. The answer is both yes and no, and we have a lot to learn from the no.

The Dolphin Among the Tigers

Educators who are fans of standardized tests are particularly fond of the Programme for International Student Assessment (PISA) tests. PISA was launched in 2000 by Paris-based Organisation for Economic Co-operation and Development (OECD). Its main objective is to evaluate educational systems by testing the knowledge of fifteen-year-old students in more than seventy participating countries, and then comparing the results. PISA tests are conducted once every three years, and the results are often used by governments to improve local educational standards. If you're curious whether French kids are as good at reading as German kids, PISA can tell you. If you want to know whether Canadian kids are as good at math as American kids, PISA can tell you.

Hidden in the data, though, is something the tests weren't designed to disclose: whether authoritarian education is the best way to get students to perform to the very highest standards. A quick glance at Table 3.1 will reveal a surprising outlier among the tigers in science, reading, and mathematics.

Table 3.1 PISA Scores, 2009

Science	PISA Score	Reading	PISA Score	Mathematics	PISA Score
Shanghai, China	575	Shanghai, China	556	Shanghai, China	600
Finland	554	Korea	539	Singapore	539
Hong Kong, China	549	Finland	536	Hong Kong, China	536
Singapore	542	Hong Kong, China	533	Korea	533
Japan	539	Singapore	526	Taiwan	526

Source: OECD, *PISA 2009 Results: Executive Summary*, 2010, http://www.oecd.org/pisa/pisaproducts/46619703.pdf, Figure 1.

Finland: Navigating Towards Twenty-First-Century Success

It turns out that millions of Asian parents are right: if you drill your kids hard enough, they can rise to the top. The sleepless nights, the drudgery, the countless sacrifices—they can be expected to pay off in the end. The thing is, it turns out that students can rise to the top without the grueling regimen of memorization and endless study. You may have noticed that Finland shows up in two of the PISA tables. Finland is the astonishing outlier here, not because it's the only non-Asian country in the top five performers, but because it has an educational system that's the complete opposite of those of the authoritarian systems.

In Finland, children don't enter school until age seven, and creative play is highly encouraged, with seventy-five minutes of play per day built into the elementary program.[5] Since the Finns believe that education is a gradual process and not a competition, they don't use standardized tests to evaluate a child's progression to a higher grade. Children have little homework, and the few tests they have don't start until mid-teenage years. The only standardized test (the National Matriculation Exam at age sixteen) is taken at the end of upper secondary school. Finnish students do partake in other types of "tests," though. In these tests, they're asked simple questions to evaluate the effectiveness of teachers and the school they're in. Teachers are well-educated (most have a master's degree) and are highly respected in Finnish society.

So, how did a country with such a relaxed approach to education do so well in the PISA tests? This question intrigued educators from around the world, and a number of them made a beeline to Finland to study its educational model. Here's what they were told by the Finnish government: "To preserve knowledge based education and economies, a country has to prepare not just some of its population well, but its entire population well, for the new economy."[6] In Finland, the main driver of educational policy is cooperation, not competition. Also, students are never separated into "streams" based on greater or lesser academic aptitude, and all schools are equal. No private schools or school rankings are part of the system.

It's not hard to see that the Finnish educational model works to create an internal locus of control in its students. Students learn that their interests matter and that they're unique individuals, yet still part of a group.

The Finnish government spends 30 percent *less* on each student than does the United States.[7] As well, the difference between the weakest and strongest student is smallest in Finland than other countries, and Finland ranks consistently in the PISA top five without the pain and suffering seen among its Asian country cohorts. The Finnish educational system is simpler, easier, cheaper, and far healthier than the tiger systems. The system works because it's in sync with how humans truly learn and yearn to live: through a balanced life that values play, exploration, social connection, and collaboration.

If you're concerned that the Finnish model doesn't hold up in the world we live in, take a look at how many Nobel Prize winners have come out of each of the countries listed in Table 3.1 per ten million people. All five prizes (Chemistry, Literature, Peace, Physics, and Physiology or Medicine) and the Nobel Memorial Prize in Economic Sciences are considered in the following list:

- China: 0.06
- Finland: 7.6
- Hong Kong: 1.39
- Japan: 1.49
- Singapore: 0
- South Korea: 0.205
- Taiwan: 0.43

If we just compare South Korea and Finland in terms of Nobel Laureates per ten million people, we don't just see double or triple the number of prize winners, we see thirty-seven times the number of prize winners! Despite its consistent inclusion in the top-five PISA rankings, South Korea ranks sixty-second out of seventy-one countries for producing Nobel Prize winners. South Korean children are clearly hardworking and dedicated students, but the tiger is getting in their way. Despite its high costs in every metric such as physical health, mental health, social health, spiritual health, and financial health, tiger educational systems fail when it comes to producing the kind of creative and critical thinkers that know how to communicate their ideas and collaborate.

CQ: Essential Twenty-First-Century Skills

The unprecedented ability of companies to analyze large data pools on company performance has revolutionized hiring practices and leadership. Google has the *most* data and has been looking at it for the *longest* period of time. In June 2013, its senior vice-president of people operations said this: "One of the things we have seen from all of our data crunching is that GPAs and test scores are worthless as criteria for hiring productive and innovative employees—Google famously used to ask everyone for transcripts, GPAs, and test scores, but we don't anymore. ... We found that they don't predict anything."[8] If transcripts, GPAs, and test scores don't predict anything, what does? Google has indicated that it wants "people who are good at figuring out stuff where there is no obvious answer."[9]

To do well in today's fast-paced, highly social, ultracompetitive, and globally connected world, our children need twenty-first-century skills. Four essential twenty-first-century skills were determined by The Assessment and Teaching of 21st Century Skills (ATC21S™), an organization at the University of Melbourne that includes more than 250 researchers from sixty different institutions worldwide. These skills have been incorporated in educational institutions and workplace environments everywhere. Here they are:

- *Creativity.* Creativity has been identified by today's business leaders as the most important competency for the future.
- *Critical thinking.* It isn't knowing the "right answers" that counts, but rather knowing how to ask the "right questions."
- *Communication.* You can have all the raw intelligence in the world, but if you can't express your thoughts effectively and in different media, it won't matter.
- *Collaboration.* Whether it's in the family, the workplace, or the global community, being able to learn from and inspire others while working in a team is key in today's work world.

I refer to this set of core skills for twenty-first-century success as the *complete quotient,* or *CQ.* As you likely know, IQ (intelligence quotient) represents raw intellectual ability, and EQ (emotional quotient) represents emotional intelligence. For success in the twenty-first century, our children will need CQ as well.

The Emergence of CQ Expectations in Education and Business

Jack Andraka is the fifteen-year-old winner of Intel's International Science and Engineering Fair. Jack designed a test for cancer, which is twenty-eight times faster, twenty-eight times cheaper, and one-hundred times more sensitive than current testing methods. In a world awash in unfiltered information, the real contribution of the creative mind is not so much to remember things as to find the important connections between them. In a field as specialized as cancer research, who would think that a teenager could make such a valuable contribution? That's the power of CQ.

Jack created the initial test based on information he found through research on Google and Wikipedia. After designing the test, he needed some way to see if it worked, so he went back to the Internet. He emailed hundreds of research labs and researchers to find out whether they were interested in his invention. After about 199 rejections, he received one invitation, which is what has led him to success. Jack has made headlines around the world, and he has traveled and rubbed shoulders with political and scientific dignitaries at distinguished places such as TED Conferences, The Royal Society of Medicine in London, and even The White House.

Jack's success has less to do with nineteenth-century knowledge (such as how well he may have performed on standardized tests) and more to do with twenty-first-century smarts. His creativity and critical-thinking skills allowed him to invent his test for cancer, and his skill in collaboration and communication allowed him to successfully find a partner for it. Many students have access to Google and Wikipedia, but his self-motivation and independence inspired him to fully explore his interests. If he had been pushed into something that he didn't find interesting, we all know that this project wouldn't have ever reached this level. Jack's sincere wish to make the world a better place compelled him to push on in the face of a lot of rejection.

In 2011, Sir Richard Branson tweeted that he would fly anybody to meet him for drinks if they donated $2,000 dollars to Free the Children.[10] A nineteen-year-old named Stacey Ferreira jumped at the opportunity, and she and her older brother, Scott, were flown out to Miami with eighteen others to meet with Branson. When they made their donation, Stacey and Scott not only helped Free the Children but also seized the occasion to pitch their new business idea, MySocialCloud, in a brief meeting with Branson. The siblings then returned to California and kept in touch with Branson via email and Twitter. Soon Branson introduced the siblings to his friend Jerry Murdock, the co-founder of a venture capital firm in New York. Murdock eventually visited the Ferreiras' office in Los Angeles. The next day, Murdock announced that he and Branson would invest a million dollars in MySocialCloud.

A few months later, from her dorm room at New York University, Stacey Ferreira was overseeing all marketing efforts, coordinating conference calls with her diverse group of programmers, managing strategic operations, evaluating user experience, and streamlining the MySocialCloud vision. Scott became the chief executive officer of MySocialCloud while attending the University of Southern California, working towards his bachelor degree in architecture.

Scott and Stacey's story would have been rare ten years ago and almost unheard of twenty years ago, when virtually no easy opportunities existed to meet with people in powerful positions. Through avenues such as social media, the twenty-first century is opening up these kinds of opportunities like never before. And those with CQ will come out on top.

Today, businesses and universities are competing to attract the Jack Andrakas and the Stacey and Scott Ferreiras out there. The twenty-first-century world offers diverse opportunities completely outside the narrow nineteenth-century pathways to "success." As a result, the narrow nineteenth-century pathways are quickly becoming obsolete. In a conversation I had with a career counselor at one of India's leading universities, I was told that "there are far more demands and opportunities now than ever before for graduates. You don't just have to be a doctor, lawyer, or engineer anymore to get a good job. But if you are, you better be able to innovate and think on your feet. There are new jobs popping up every day, and technology has been the main reason for this. Over the next 10 years, grades will matter less, and innovation and communication will be key." The time is ripe for young people to employ CQ on their own, and those who do will be the ones to succeed. In order to survive, universities and businesses have realized that they need to adapt and create environments that foster CQ. This new reality is helping shift the focus of admissions and interviewing processes at universities and businesses everywhere.

The University of British Columbia (UBC) became Canada's first major university to incorporate non-academic criteria into its admissions process. As UBC's associate vice-president and registrar noted: "We were increasingly realizing we were missing elements of that student's experience and accomplishments. Even the challenges they face can be powerful predictors of the future roles they may fill."[11] Students who applied to UBC for entrance into the 2012–13 year were asked to complete a five-question survey, which had them share personal and meaningful experiences.

Along the same lines, in response to complaints from the business community that its graduates often lacked vital leadership and interpersonal skills, UBC's Sauder School of Business changed its admissions policy in 2004 to include broader-based criteria beyond GPAs and test scores. As a result, those complaints dropped dramatically and, to the school's benefit, it also attracted students interested in broader extracurricular activities, such as student government.[12]

Harvard Business School has a program called the 2+2 Program. Young people accepted into the program spend two years pursuing work opportunities of interest to them followed by two years in the Harvard Business School master's program. Students have access to a mentor, but otherwise have complete freedom to play, explore, connect, and collaborate as they like during the first two years. Now, why would Harvard have such a program? The program gives students the opportunity to follow their passion and curiosity while developing exceptional twenty-first-century skills through hands-on, unstructured learning. These students bring their CQ, innovative thinking, and real-life experiences back into the classroom to the benefit of other students and the business school overall. It's a win-win situation for everyone.

As a doctor and an instructor to medical students, I'm delighted to see that medical schools too are moving towards greater emphasis on CQ. And for good reason: far too many patients have been treated by "smart" doctors who lack empathy, communication skills, and the ability to think creatively. We all want doctors who can critically analyze the endless data available and then appropriately apply that data to real-life situations. As we saw with Tom in the previous chapter, the tiger model just doesn't prepare young people to become that kind of doctor.

Today, many applicants to medical school, law school, business school, and other graduate schools are interviewed by a panel of admissions officers and human resources personnel to observe their ability to communicate, collaborate, and think critically. Individual interviews are painstakingly and profession-ally designed to elicit responses that reflect empathy, creativity, ethics, and problem solving—or a lack thereof.

The Medical College Admissions Test (MCAT) is set to change dramatically by 2015. Among the changes are questions connecting the basic sciences of human behavior and thought. As well, the MCAT will include a new section that doesn't require specific knowledge but will be used to test reasoning and critical analysis.[13]

Even the Scholastic Aptitude Test (SAT), which is essential for admission to US colleges, has changed. In 2001, the president of the University of California (UC) criticized the SAT for some sections that test knowledge only a select few students would have. He threatened to drop a part of the test when reviewing candidates for UC schools. In 2005, these concerns were addressed; certain content was dropped, and other content was added, including an essay and more critical reading questions.[14]

The profit-driven world of business seems to be moving away from the tiger model at a fast pace. Businesses around the world are in pursuit of those individuals who possess "soft skills." The Yale School of Business recently added mandatory EQ testing for its MBA applicants.[15] Tom Kolditz, director of the school's leadership development program, states, "We want students to have greater self-awareness. We want them to improve their ability to manage emotions and influence others."[16] A similar test is being used for admissions at Notre Dame's Mendoza College of Business to identify what the senior associate director of MBA admissions calls "diamonds in the rough." And Dartmouth's Tuck School of Business asks individuals providing a letter of recommendation to score an applicant's curiosity and ability to cope with pressure.[17]

Of course technical skills are important, but if employees don't have CQ, their contributions will be limited. "Soft skills tend to differentiate good college graduates from exceptional college graduates," says Joseph Krok, university research liaison at Britain's Rolls-Royce.[18] "Many technical programs around the world have historically focused more on technical depth ...

We've been communicating to universities the importance of soft skills," adds Paul McIntyre, vice-president in charge of global recruiting at British Petrol (BP).[19] One employer told the global consultancy McKinsey & Co.: "I have never fired an engineer for bad engineering, but I have fired an engineer for lack of teamwork."[20]

Even fields that used to be safe havens for those without CQ increasingly require creativity and collaboration. For example, some interviews for chartered accountant jobs at PwC have included a component where applicants were assessed on their interpersonal skills as they worked together in a cooking class. Yes, a cooking class! Jobs that involve working with other people—especially people from diverse cultures, demographics, and locations—require the skills tigers just don't have.

Now that we're shifting from a landscape where nineteenth-century tigers could flourish to one where they'll have difficulty even getting an interview, let alone making it through the real world of business or higher education, our parenting models must also shift. We know intuitively, and now see through research and data, that authoritarian systems with top-down leadership don't allow us to thrive in today's world. So why are we trying to parent according to the same old model?

A Life in Balance: The Basis for Health, Happiness, and Success

The changes we're seeing in our schools, universities, and businesses all favor a model far more in tune with what truly motivates and energizes the human mind and creates healthier, happier, and self-motivated people.

Dr. George Vaillant's famous Grant Study of Adult Development was the subject of the book *The Triumphs of*

Experience.[21] Spanning many decades, this study was the first and remains the longest and most comprehensive scientific examination of long-term adult wellness, happiness, and success of its kind. The study, which began in 1938 at Harvard University, has followed 268 male Harvard undergraduates throughout the course of their lives. The researchers measured an astounding range of psychological, anthropological, and physical traits—including IQ, major organ function, childhood behaviors such as bed-wetting, personality type, height, Rorschach inkblots interpretations, handwriting analysis, drinking habits, brain EEGs, physical looks, family background, relationships, the size of their "lip seam," and even the "hanging length of [the] scrotum"—in an effort to determine what factors contribute most strongly to human flourishing.

All subjects filled out questionnaires every two years about their everyday lives and health. Every five years, detailed data about their health was obtained from their physicians. Whenever possible, the men were personally interviewed to get more in-depth information as well as to understand their adjustment to a changing world and life. The data are still being collected today, as 30 percent of these men have lived into their nineties.

Vaillant's study has given us never-before-seen scientific insight into health, happiness, and success. Over the years, some surprising (or maybe not so surprising) trends have been identified:[22]

- *Above a certain level, intelligence doesn't matter.* There was no significant difference in maximum income earned by men with IQs in the 110–115 range and men with IQs higher than 150.
- *Adaptability is a key determinant of success.* Mature adaptive style was the personality trait that by age fifty was

an excellent predictor of those who would be in the "happy-well" group (that is, those with good subjective and objective mental and physical health)—which represents the top quartile of the Harvard men studied. Vaillant described the mature adaptive style as being able to "make a lemon into lemonade," which to me means being able to adapt creatively and positively to any situation. Vaillant also stated that the use of altruism and a sense of humor in handling conflict and stress were features of this mature adaptive style.

- *Six factors are important predictors of those who would reach the "happy-well" group.* In addition to a mature adaptive style, six factors predicted membership in the "happy-well" group: no smoking, little use of alcohol, regular exercise, maintenance of normal weight, and a stable marriage.

- *The warmth of one's relationships has a powerful effect on health, happiness, and success.* For example, the men who scored highest on measurements of "warm relationships" earned an average of $141,000 a year more at their peak salaries (usually between ages fifty-five and sixty) than the men who scored lowest. These men not only had better financial success but also were three times more likely to be included in *Who's Who* lists for their professional success. Moreover, men who had "warm" childhood relationships with their mothers (remember, the study began in 1938) earned an average of $87,000 more a year than men whose mothers were uncaring. In contrast, men who had poor childhood relationships with their mothers were much more likely to develop dementia when old. Vaillant's key takeaway, in his own words, is this: "The seventy-five years and twenty million dollars expended on the Grant Study points ... to a straightforward five-word conclusion: 'Happiness is love. Full stop.'"[23]

This all sounds great, but how can we actually go about becoming "happy-well"? Simple: doing leads to being. By adapting, we become adaptable. By performing acts of altruism, we become altruistic. By being warm and empathic, we become connected with others. We need to *do* all of these things because it makes us *become* all of these things. However, our actions shape our internal character only when we act according to our true intentions. Vaillant's study and numerous others on happiness, success, failure, and motivation all confirm the same thing: health comes first, happiness is love and connection, and success requires adaptability. To be "happy-well," we must tame the imbalanced tiger in us and instead embrace our inner, balanced dolphin.

Why Dolphins?

Why the dolphin way, you might ask? Why not the dog way? The walrus way? The fruit fly way? Dolphins have a number of attributes that combine to make them a powerful metaphor for successful living in this complicated world. That said, nothing is wrong with tigers! The tiger–dolphin comparison is not a judgment of the animals themselves, any more than "The Tortoise and the Hare" is about how terrible hares are. What we understand about the story is not that hares have a troubling tendency to boast and be overconfident about their talents— it's that *we* do. We don't come away with a new respect for tortoises—we pause for a moment and realize that if we're faced with a challenge, we must remain calm, persistent, and steady. In other words, it's not really about the animals, it's about us. Still, in this sense, the tiger is not so unlike the hare, and the dolphin has certain similarities with the tortoise. I can guarantee you that it's more fun to be a dolphin.

Humans have had a long love affair with dolphins. Maybe it's because the dolphin is widely accepted as one of the world's most intelligent animals. The dolphin brain is uniquely large. In relative size, it's second only to the human brain and four times the size of a chimpanzee's. Brain size is correlated with intelligence, creativity, learning, communication, and social connection, and dolphins display all of these qualities with gusto. Dolphins are also well known for being joyful and clever. They're true social creatures, traveling and living in pods. They teach their young through role modeling, play, and guidance. What many don't know is that dolphins are considered among the world's most altruistic and collaborative animal species. Helping one another and their communities is a core feature of their existence.

The dolphin parenting model is about guiding rather than directing, encouraging rather than instructing, and teaching by example. The dolphin way of life is about emphasizing the importance of play, exploration, social bonds, altruism, contribution, and family and community values. Of course, all of these attributes are also natural to human parenting. Because of our fearful and imbalanced lives full of overgathering, over-competing, and overprotecting, it's helpful to look outside our species to remind ourselves what it means to live a balanced life. I consider the terms *dolphin parenting*, *balanced parenting*, and *intuitive parenting* to be interchangeable. Dolphin parenting simply asks you to act on what you already know as a balanced and intuitive human being.

The Dolphin: A Model of Health, Happiness, and Success

So, how exactly can the dolphin point the way to parenting that can truly equip our children on their journey through the ever-changing waters of the twenty-first century? For one thing, dolphins exhibit the same essential skills necessary for twenty-first-century success. They have CQ!

- *Creativity*. They create "tools" to hunt and find food, such as using sea sponges over their snouts to forage for food on the ocean floor.
- *Critical thinking*. They can recognize and work around many kinds of problems, such as fishing traps.
- *Communication*. Many scientists equate their system of communication through whistles, squeaks, and physical gestures to actual language.
- *Collaboration*. They are highly social and hunt, play, and live all aspects of life in a pod.

Dolphins aren't on the prowl all the time nor are they constantly competing with one another. They play, explore, sleep, exercise, bond socially, and contribute as well. They seem to have individual interests—some play with seaweed, some body-surf coastal swells for fun, and some play-fight with other dolphins. They even engage in complex play behaviors such as making and diving through bubble rings. Dolphins have strong social bonds with their family members and with other members of their pod. They even exhibit "friendship" with other dolphins who share common behaviors.

Dolphins are self-reliant yet socially connected. They live and raise their young in ways we would describe as ethical; their habit of helping one another and other species seems altruistic. They have been known to protect humans from shark attacks and to rescue beached whales—actions that show responsibility to and compassion for those outside their pod and even outside their species.

Also, did you know that the top of the ocean's food chain—the killer whale, or orca—is actually a dolphin?! The orca is the world's most powerful top-level predator. But unlike solitary hunters such as tigers, sharks, and polar bears, orcas are highly social and collaborative, making them all the more powerful.

Dolphins know the world can be a competitive and dangerous place, and that's why they band together. An orca can easily kill a shark, but other dolphins work together when it comes to dealing with predators. I like to think of dolphins as the Finns (no pun intended) of the ocean world—on top not because they're the most competitive, but because they're creative, playful, and can work well with others.

Dolphins are also wonderfully adaptable. In terms of their behavior, they can form long-term associations with other species (such as tuna, sea turtles, and humans) and adapt to feed on available local prey. Previously independent pods have even been known to unite to hunt for new food sources together.[24] In terms of their physical adaptations, while most dolphins live in saltwater, some of the species can live in freshwater. Dolphins are also streamlined so that they can move fast (up to one hundred miles per hour) to catch prey and escape predators. As well, their eyeballs move independently from each other so that one can look straight ahead for prey while the other looks around for predators.

Humans, too, must adapt as we face the changing world of the twenty-first century. Parents are under great pressure and our children are too. With traits of adaptability, a healthy lifestyle, altruism, and sociability, the dolphin would certainly have come out on top of Vaillant's study! As parents, if we can adapt and nurture these traits in our children, they too can be healthy, happy, and successful at home, in the classroom, in the board-room, and in the community.

A Dolphin's Self-Motivation and CQ

Charlotte, a student, contacted me by phone and left a message asking if she could do some volunteer research on the issue of substance use in young adults. Oddly enough, Charlotte wasn't interested in applying to medical school like most students who contact me; she was an undergraduate interested in law. At the time, I already had enough students to supervise, and didn't really want to take on more. However, the enthusiasm with which Charlotte communicated her unique request piqued my interest, and I called her back. Within seconds of being on the phone with her, I was drawn in by her positive energy. Within minutes, I was sold by her creative ideas, which she spelled out brilliantly in a short time frame. She wanted to research the issue of the legal drinking age in Canada (nineteen) versus the United States (twenty-one) and how that may impact drinking on college and university campuses. Although I loved the idea, I saw some obstacles to this research, which I brought forth. Charlotte quickly problem solved those obstacles right there on phone. I was still unsure about taking on another student, especially someone so young. She must have picked this up in my tone, because she immediately discussed how this project would be a win-win for everyone. She already had a law journal picked out that she wanted to submit her research to (an obvious plus for both of us, but also for numerous stakeholders—policy makers, police, health professionals, and campus administrators). Within a ten-minute phone call, Charlotte's display of creative and critical thinking, communication and collaboration skills, and her positive energy and clear desire to lead a project that would be good for herself and the world made it impossible for me to say no to her! She was a total dolphin.

Yes, Charlotte was a highly ambitious dolphin, but the difference between her and an ambitious tiger is worlds apart. First, she could think on her feet—I don't see these traits in individuals who have been brought up overscheduled, overinstructed, and overmanaged. Her *own* passion and internal drive for learning was clear. I felt that I could count on her to be independent yet still part of a team. She was not a crispie or a teacup—she seemed happy with where she was in life yet had a clear vision for her future, which made her likeable and pleasant to be around. Finally, she seemed trustworthy, respectful, and fair—which is what makes for a true leader.

I knew Charlotte was applying to law school. Her top choice was Stanford Law School, one of the hardest law schools to get into in the world! Because my interactions with her were so pleasant and productive, I felt bonded to her and wanted to help her pursue her (not her parents') personal interest, for which she had so much enthusiasm. Before she even asked me for a reference letter, I offered her one. I also connected her with my brother who went to Stanford and also law school in California. Because she's so likeable, he jumped on board as a mentor too. I prioritized some of our joint research projects so that she could present the scientific findings she had worked so hard for at a national conference—a great résumé item for her application. When it came to writing the Stanford reference, I was asked to assess Charlotte on areas such as creativity, communication, critical thinking, and collaboration. The final lines in my letter were these: "In over ten years of teaching and supervising under-graduate and graduate students, Charlotte ranks among the top 1 percent of all students I have come across as she has developed exceptional key twenty-first-century skills. Charlotte's proven success is just the beginning of her story as she has powerful self-motivation to further pursue her deep personal passion of law and contribution to her community—whether that of Stanford or the greater world." A few months ago, I got a lovely email from an exuberant Charlotte who just got in to Stanford Law School. I was happy for Charlotte, but whether or not she had been accepted to Stanford Law School, I have no doubt Charlotte has what it takes to be successful.

Whether children parented by dolphins get into a top college or find their own path that may or may not include school, they are able to leave the pod, venture out on their own, come back if they choose, and eventually create their own pods.

If the thought of a "CQ tutor," "adaptability coach," or "balance camp" has crossed your mind, I'm begging you to forget all that! The great news is that it's in our nature to thrive and fairly simple to achieve these dolphin attributes—as long as we get rid of the tiger lurking inside us. Let's take a closer look at how dolphins achieve all of this for their young, themselves, and their pods, and have fun doing it!

Chapter 4

. . . .

HOW DO DOLPHINS THRIVE?

When I met my children's pediatrician, Dr. Chow, I was struck by how great he was with children. He's incredibly bright and ambitious, but I was most impressed with his creativity. He used a straw to entertain my child and measure his head circumference at the same time, to take just one example. When I asked about his background (before I got out of my obsessive need for this kind of information), I expected to hear about his elite education. I was shocked when he told me he grew up on a goat farm in a small town in Indonesia and barely attended school until age ten! (Of course, now, after all the research for this book, I wouldn't be shocked at all.)

We both came from non-tiger backgrounds, but when I met Dr. Chow, he had something I didn't yet have: the ability to work intuitively. He never pushed his patients or their parents regarding what to do. Instead, he seemed to be able to get them to realize what needed to be done themselves, and he had an authenticity and genuineness that made you want to be around him and listen to what he had to say. Dr. Chow appeared to be loved by everyone that walked into his office. He also seemed to be able to adapt to whomever walked through his door.

In over ten years of working with highly diverse patients with highly diverse problems, I quickly found that no one approach worked with every person or even with the same person in every situation. Then I had my own three children and realized that the same applied to my parenting: each of my children needed something different and at different times. Both as a doctor and a parent, I, too, had to constantly adapt to the person and issues at hand. For me, the process of becoming as intuitive and adaptable as Dr. Chow included three crucial steps: (1) I had to identify and stick to my true intentions, (2) I had to guide instead of instruct, and (3) I had to do both while being genuine in every way—which meant I had to know my values and be true to them, no matter what.

I had been a doctor for about eight years before I became a parent. Once I became a parent, I found that my doctor role made me a better parent, and vice versa. Doctors want to help their patients, and parents want to help their children. I had the good intention of wanting to help my patients and my children, but it was distorted by the negative influences around me. As a parent, I was affected by the fear associated with the pressures of parenting in the twenty-first century. As a doctor, I was also affected by fear—fear of missing a diagnosis, of being disliked by my patients, of being named in a lawsuit. I had to make a fundamental shift in my thinking in order to make a fundamental shift in my actions. I had to realize that I had the choice. I also had to go back to my original intentions for wanting to become a doctor and a parent. As a doctor, I had to reassert my personal commitment to always act in a way that would help my patients achieve better health. *That* is my job—as opposed to relieving their anxiety, avoiding a lawsuit, or becoming their friends. Once

I reconnected with my intentions, I found I could communicate with my patients much more easily.

When I applied this knowledge to my parenting, it helped me immensely. Once I clearly identified and stayed true to my intentions as a parent—to raise a child who thrives in all aspects of life, not just one narrow path (such as getting into a certain school or becoming my best friend)—things became much easier. I could make decisions without an immense struggle, and I felt a lot less stress.

Once my intentions became top of mind, I thought I was set. But I wasn't always effective in the execution of my intentions. I was often *telling* my patients and children what to do rather than *guiding* them to the desire to carry out the action themselves. For example, most doctors want their patients to adopt a healthy lifestyle—to stop smoking, eat better, exercise more. Yet how many actually help their patients achieve that? In fact, one may say modern medicine is failing when you consider that modifiable lifestyle diseases such as obesity, diabetes, heart disease, and addictions are killing more people now than ever before.

That was one of my first insights as a doctor. Many, if not all, of my patients were suffering from unhealthy lifestyles consisting of too little sleep and exercise, and too much stress and busyness. In response, I researched how I could best help them change their lifestyles. What I found was that telling someone what to do only worked for about 20 percent or less of patients—those who were already prepared to make a change. That means 80 percent of patients were in a different "stage of change," often called the precontemplation stage (that is, denial or not knowing) or the contemplation stage (that is, knowing but not acting). (See Chapter 9 for more on the stages of change.) So, for doctors, directing and instructing the majority of people is completely ineffective. Saying to a patient, "Stop smoking, lose weight, sleep better, or exercise more" simply doesn't work. The same is true for parents. Saying to children, "Stop fooling around, pay attention, try harder, and change your attitude" simply doesn't work.

What does work for both parents and doctors is *guiding*. Guiding is the balance between instruction and no instruction, between direction and no direction, between authoritarian and permissive, between the tiger and the jellyfish. Guiding can come in a number of forms: through advice, a range of proposed solutions, or sometimes just waiting for someone to figure things out on their own; but it *always* needs to be done in a relationship that feels supportive. Guiding is also the basis for the most effective and inspiring human-to-human interaction, whether you are a parent, coach, teacher, employer, manager, or anyone who works with other people. Pushing, directing, hovering, bribing, pleading, cajoling—even when combined—can't come close to the positive outcomes associated with guiding.

Once I started applying the guiding method to my practice and my parenting, I said to myself, *OK I now have the right intentions AND the right method, I'm set.* Wrong. While my methods would work for some patients and some problems, they wouldn't work for all patients and all problems. Since I was one of the few physicians around who specialized in youth addiction and motivation, I was seeing increasingly complex cases with tougher and tougher teenagers and their parents. At times, I was becoming exhausted and skeptical of my methods. I could win over some of the tough teenagers, but not all of them. Early in my career, I'll never forget when an angry fifteen-year-old boy whom I had been seeing for a few months said to me, "Dr. Kang, you are a joke and a waste of time. My neighbor who just moved in two weeks ago has helped me more by playing street hockey with me than you ever have." My response was mixed to say the least. It was wonderful news for my young patient who seemed to have a breakthrough experience, but I couldn't help but feel a sort of defeat.

Once again, I searched for the answer to what really influenced people, outside the confines of a doctor's office. More research led to an answer that was both earth-shattering and completely predictable at the same time. What I found was a truth that applies to human interaction that I intuitively knew but had buried under all my scientific techniques. It's as simple as this: who we are on the inside is the most powerful predictor of our ability to motivate others. The most effective individuals— parents, therapists, teachers, coaches, and mentors that effectively change other people's lives—all have the same qualities. Regardless of how much training they have, what university they went to, or how many degrees they've earned, their authenticity, empathy, and kindness led to their effectiveness. For me, this was good and bad news. I felt genuine, kind, and empathic, but I was still not scoring 100 percent with my intention to help all my patients, especially the tough teenagers!

In an effort to create a stronger link between my authentic self and my actions, I started showing my patients more empathy, making small gestures of kindness, smiling more, making real eye contact, and making more time for what mattered to them instead of what was on my agenda. I made a commitment to be authentic and never say anything I didn't believe in because that's a death trap, especially with teenagers who can see right through fakeness even if you have the right intention and method. For example, I finally admitted to an angry fifteen-year-old boy (and myself) that his school (one of "the best") was a mismatch for his nature. His school was too rigid and structured for his personality, and he was right that everyone's denial of this reality was slowly "ruining" his life. Once I put myself in his shoes, I could see how he felt imprisoned by a system that was stifling him and how angry he was that no one noticed or acknowledged his plight. I was able to express empathy for his dilemma kindly and genuinely because I believed it inside, even though his parents became angry with me for saying so. My empathy didn't lead him to give up on school, as his parents feared. It actually motivated him to jump through the required hoops to get his diploma because he finally felt understood. My empathy actually freed him from the vicious cycle of trying to prove he was right. Not only did my actions help me show genuineness, kindness, and empathy more, they helped me become more genuine, kind, and empathic.

The same goes for parenting. I've heard many teenagers say, "Yeah, my parents might love me, but I don't think they like me or even really know me." The parents in these cases may not have been demonstrating their empathy to their children. Children can only experience the parental behaviors we show them—not what's in our hearts and minds and not our true intentions. Some parents feel they must show no cracks in their tough veneer of authority, and others feel they must show no imperfections. However, by never showing their deep fears, worries, and weaknesses, they're sending the message that these things aren't appropriate or even a normal part of life. When we fail to be genuine, we create a distance between ourselves and our children.

The Benefits of Authoritative Parenting

Dolphin parenting is much more than a style of parenting. If you're reading this book, you likely believe that parenting isn't just about ensuring children are well behaved, have high marks at school, or even have a strong bond with their parents. It's about raising children who will have a healthy relationship with the world—with their community, workplace, spouse, siblings, children, parents, and, most important, themselves. It's also about raising children who will become an integral part of their world, experience the ups and downs of a life with grace, and make the most of their limited time on this earth. Finally, it's about raising children who can meet challenges with determination and hard work, be driven by their passions and talents, be proud of their accomplishments, bounce back from hardship, and find a balance in body, mind, and soul. The dolphin way is a philosophy, a way of life. It's not only a method for how to do things with your child but also a way of being with your child—and living your own life. Rather than focusing on turning your child into something, it's about bringing out what's already there—in your child and in you.

Because the dolphin way is intuitive, it's *not* something completely new that we have to learn. It's simply something we have to reawaken within ourselves or bring our awareness back to.

Back in Chapter 1, I discussed two styles of maladaptive parenting: authoritarian parenting (the tiger) and permissive parenting (the jellyfish). Choosing to parent like the dolphin is easy when you think of the numerous and serious drawbacks of authoritarian and permissive parenting. The style of parenting that finds a perfect balance between the two is called *authoritative parenting* (yes—the term is confusingly close to *authoritarian*), and it's the style at the heart of the dolphin way.

It should come as no surprise that in the authoritative dolphin style of parenting, the parent is a clear authority figure (not a friend, personal assistant, helicopter, slave, or slave driver). Dolphin parents establish clear rules and guidelines as they nurture their children, reason with their children, and respond to their children's emotional needs (versus demanding, cajoling, bribing, and imposing). Their idea of discipline is being assertive rather than restrictive and being supportive rather than punishing or dismissive. Unlike permissive jellyfish parents, dolphin parents enforce rules and don't let their children get away with bad behavior. Unlike authoritarian tiger parents, dolphin parents show plenty of warmth and communicate the reasons behind rules.

Authoritative dolphin parenting has its benefits:

- Being warm and responsive helps children form secure attachments and protects them from internalizing issues such as depression and anxiety.
- Enforcing limits decreases the chance children will engage in acting out behaviors such as aggression, interpersonal conflict, and drug and alcohol abuse.
- Communicating about thoughts and feelings strengthens children's empathy, emotional regulation, and relationship skills.
- Showing understanding for academic struggles helps children become better problem solvers and learners.
- Encouraging independence helps children develop self-reliance, a desire to help others, and better emotional health.

Studies of different parenting styles consistently show that authoritative parenting offers the most positive results for children and parents.[1] Children raised by authoritative parents report less depression and anxiety, have better self-esteem, are rated more "prosocial" and kind, and have an improved quality of life than children raised by authoritarian or permissive parents. A US study showed that undergraduate children with authoritative parents said that their parents had a greater influence on them than their peers.[2] Guess what else? The authoritative style is most beneficial when the entire community operates in this way!

Keeping a balance between being an authoritarian tiger and a permissive jellyfish can be challenging, but authoritative parenting is central to successful dolphin parenting. The good news is that the dolphin way doesn't just bring balance to the parent–child relationship, it brings balance to all aspects of life. And it's only through maintaining balance that we thrive.

The Art and Science of Creating a Balanced Life

Mother Nature rewards us for acting on our intuition. These rewards come in the form of complex neurochemical interactions. For example, when the neurochemical dopamine is released, it immediately fills us with a sense of well-being or joy. When we take an action and then experience the rewards of dopamine, we're internally driven to do whatever we did again. This is the basis of our brain's positive feedback loop, which goes kind of like this: *Do something good for your survival > receive positive reward via dopamine pathways > feel well-being or joy > gain the self-motivation to do something good for your survival again.*

Since species survival is the motivation for our biological processes, this feedback loop keeps us healthy and able to reproduce. Just to be clear: I'm not talking about actions that unnaturally activate dopamine, such as drugs and alcohol. Some people turn to these substances when their natural dopamine releasers are *out* of balance, which means they've ceased to act properly. The reason these substances can be so dangerous is that they override our intuition for our own health and force dopamine activation unnaturally. For example, cocaine releases whopping amounts of dopamine, thus hijacking natural neurochemical processes that help us figure out how to live.

These feedback loops also work if you do something negative. In that case, the loop looks kind of like this: *Do something bad for your survival > receive neurochemical signals such as fatigue, stress, and hunger > feel crappy > understand the signal to change your behavior > do something good for your survival > receive positive reward via dopamine pathways > feel well-being or joy.* But these systems work only if we listen to what nature is telling us. If we ignore the signals, we feel worse and worse until finally we have a serious problem that threatens our very survival.

Our job as parents becomes so much easier when we can help our children stay connected to their own biology and positive feedback loops. Balance and self-motivation are innate. That's right—we're all born with a sense of balance and naturally motivated towards health and happiness. We're generally not born with diabetes, obesity, or high cholesterol. Nor are we born depressed, anxious, apathetic, or unmotivated. Most babies, even those with life-threatening medical conditions such as congenital heart disease, show natural joy, love, and curiosity. At times, children appear to glow from the inside with something I can only describe as vitality and spirit. This light is undeniable in all children—we've all seen it in our own and in children everywhere.

This light is sometimes harder to see in adults, but it's usually still there. As adults, we see and feel it when we're playing with our children, fully immersed in music or sport, or taking in the majesty of nature. Animals also seem to exude this light, which may be why we love our pets so much. If you've ever watched a dog running in an open field with the wind blowing in his face, you know what I'm talking about.

So what happens to that light? Year after year, I've seen the inner light of child after child and patient after patient flicker, falter, and sometimes die. I've asked myself, *Is the light within our children supposed to die? Is this the normal course of human life?* My initial thoughts were, *Well, we can't stay children forever; it's natural to grow up.* But does growing up really require us to lose our vitality and spirit for life? Certainly, not all children or teenagers lose their vitality for life. Many maintain it, and many more are gaining vitality as they become older. How can one explain this? Those whose light shines brightly seem to exude a sense of balance along with traits such as confidence, curiosity, connection, creativity, and independence. Those whose light is diminishing show a life of imbalance filled with fear, anxiety, apathy, disconnection, depression, self-loathing, and hatred.

Although complex, the cause of many common health conditions, such as anxiety, depression, and addiction, is an imbalance in the interaction between one's genetics and the environment (the same is true for diabetes, obesity, and heart disease). We can't change our genetics (yet), but we can change our environment. If we change our environment, we can change our risk for and prevalence of these illnesses. The less exposure to a toxic lifestyle and the more exposure to a healthy lifestyle—especially early in life—the better. Once you recover from diseases such as diabetes, heart disease, or mental illness, if you continue to expose yourself to known lifestyle toxins, you're more likely to relapse. For example, exposure to sugar for those with diabetes, cholesterol for those with heart disease, and sleep deprivation for those with mental illness all lead to a higher chance of relapse. With lifestyle-related diseases on the rise in developing countries, an imbalanced lifestyle may be the single greatest threat humankind has ever known. But, believe it or not, it's a threat that's simple to combat—but remember, simple doesn't mean easy.

The key to treating lifestyle diseases is this: First, manage the acute dysregulation to eliminate further risk (which could include interventions such as medications, surgery, or rehab). Then, add knowledge (via education and therapy) on how to build the right skills to change the lifestyle towards more balance. Once stabilized with the right skills, one can return to the positive feedback loop we were all born to follow, but now with more connection to the signals coming our way. That's a lot better than just treating illness. Again, simple, but not necessarily easy.

I don't mean to suggest that we, alone, cause our illnesses. Even though all humans are vulnerable to lifestyle diseases, some inherit a greater risk of one or the other and thus will be more likely to manifest that illness than others with the same lifestyle. In addition, people can easily lose their health and vitality for myriad other reasons. Sometimes a traumatic event such as childhood abuse or the death of a loved one will throw someone off balance. Sometimes the trigger is a horrible boss or teacher. Very often, life's daily stresses are enough to knock us off balance. A happy childhood helps develop a strong core, but even those with a strong core can fall over if they're struck too hard. Our lifestyles, our minds, and our bodies are all intricately connected: we have to look for, pay attention to, and listen—really listen—to the cues our biology gives us because a little neglect can be all it takes to weaken our body and mind and allow us to fall. Across numerous areas of medicine, such as psychiatry, cardiology, and endocrinology, lifestyle imbalance has become the fastest-growing factor for the presentation of disease.

As parents, it's our responsibility to help our children build a solid core of strength and flexibility through a balanced lifestyle. Dolphins instinctively raise their children so that they develop these very qualities. Dolphins don't force their calves to do anything; they guide them in the right direction. Dolphins let their calves experience the natural consequences of their mistakes so they can learn from them. Dolphins create safety nets to keep their calves from harm, but they still give them a lot of chances to self-correct. Dolphins are kind and generous most of the time, but they have limits as to how much they will tolerate. By following their intuition, dolphins and their calves are able to hear Mother Nature far more clearly than we do. They don't fight against their own biology. As a result, they're rarely out of balance in the way we humans are.

Dolphins don't just follow their intuition to eat, sleep, and exercise better than many humans, they follow their natural intuition for all aspects of daily life. Humans, especially tiger parents, are seriously deficient in this area. Beyond the basics of survival, humans are heavily rewarded for other—perhaps surprising—activities. Contrary to some beliefs, these activities are not "luxuries" but necessary for our very survival, otherwise they wouldn't cause the release of the powerful neurochemicals of reward. These activities are also essential to adapting and thriving. They boost our CQ, enhance our sense of happiness, and energize our self-motivation. Participating in the following activities will tame the tiger and help bring balance to our lives:

- Playing freely
- Exploring bravely
- Bonding socially
- Contributing wholeheartedly

The good news is that we're naturally wired to pursue these activities because they reward us with health, self-motivation, well-being, joy, and vitality. *Vitality* is the capacity for continuation of a meaningful or purposeful existence.[3] It's the power to live and grow. Vitality is not something available only for the lucky few—we all have it in us.

The bad news is that if we ignore Mother Nature's guidance and don't pursue these activities, we'll find ourselves off balance, and it will be only a matter of time before we fall over and get hurt. Our vitality, then our well-being, joy, self-motivation, and our health will slip away.

So, any skeptics? If so, simply ask yourself, what makes you feel well-being and joy naturally? What activities in your day or life uplift your mood in a natural way? If not apparent at first glance, after some reflection, you'll agree that the activities in the previous list bring a sense of well-being or joy to your life. Did you notice I said "well-being" and "joy" and not "good feeling"? You can feel good from going shopping, having a glass of wine, or eating a piece of chocolate cake. I mean well-being and joy in the sense of something that lasts more than a few minutes or hours. Something that, when you think *back* on it, brings a smile to your face without guilt or regret (see how shopping, alcohol, and cake don't work?). In essence, when you feel well-being or joy, your brain is giving you natural clues about what you're meant to do. I say this with no doubt whatsoever, because these conclusions are simply based on human biology. Listen to those clues and you'll become the person you're meant to be. It's through what we do that we become who we are.

True Success: Based on Balance and High Expectations

You might look at the list in the preceding section and say, "My kids can't spend time playing, exploring, bonding socially, or contributing if they want to be successful." You might think play and contribution are unimportant and want to skip those parts of the book to find out how to get your child into a top-tier university. If so, skipping those parts of the book is the last thing you'll want to do. In those pages, you'll find out what leads to a solid internal locus of control and what truly internally motivates people towards all aspects of success.

Some may think career or financial "success" only comes from imbalance. They point to all those workaholics who are at the top of their fields and got there by scrimping on sleep, play, friendship, and altruism. Unfortunately, for many of these people, "success" really doesn't feel so successful. That's why we see so many troubles and disease among this group—including depression, anxiety, heart disease, corruption, addiction, suicide, and early death.

Thankfully, another group of successful people exists who truly encompass the meaning of the word. We may sometimes hear about their exceptional talents and contribution, but little else, as they quietly go about their lives just being great. This group achieves true success not by imbalance but by strict adherence to balance—no matter what else may be happening in their lives. The best of the best are balanced— they sleep, exercise, play, explore, bond socially, contribute, and are self-motivated.

It's not hard to see how tiger parents actually have low expectations of their children. They're not helping their children strive for success in all aspects of the meaning of the word. Tiger parents compromise the very pinnacle of what humans can achieve. Our children have the wonderful opportunity to achieve vitality and joy in life. But tiger parents settle for much less. That's not a mistake dolphins make.

Ready, Set, Go!

Now that we fully understand the dilemmas of twenty-first-century parents and have recognized a better approach, let's dive deeper into the waters of the dolphin way.

The good news is that we can certainly change what we do, how we parent, and even who we are—regardless of how old we are, how we grew up, or how ingrained our habits are. The belief that the adult brain can change in form and function has been part of science for over 120 years, but the evidence of neuroplasticity is more recent and indisputable.

We have over a trillion possible neuronal connections in our brains. Some of these connections are wired into habits—both positive and negative—and others are wired into both beneficial and self-limiting beliefs. And countless connections have not even occurred yet—their existence is pure potential. That is, the brain can form fresh pathways when neurons fire at the same time repeatedly, causing chemical changes to occur that connect them more strongly. Just like a trail through the forest becomes well-worn and easier to navigate the more it's used, our neural tracks develop the more they're used. When we repeat certain behaviors, the corresponding neural pathways develop more dendritic connections (the path becomes wider) and become more myelinated (the path becomes smoother). That's what our habits and behaviors are—the results of neural tracks that have been laid down and used over time. When we act differently, we *become* different. Wherever we put our energies is where we will develop. Neuroplasticity provides hope for change and a better life.

So let's begin our journey of change. First, we'll cover the basics of survival that provide a strong foundation for life. Then, we'll explore other areas in which tigers are seriously lacking for twenty-first-century success. Once we have the right lifestyle covered, we'll take a closer look at a dolphin parenting toolkit that features additional guidance on parenting in an authoritative way. Then we'll review a universal goal of parenting and life—self-motivation. Finally, we'll consider what happens to children who grow up the dolphin way, with your own intuition as your parental guide.

Throughout this journey, we'll be reconnecting with our intuition and adapting. I'll guide you through the transformation from the overdoing and underparenting of the tiger parent to the guiding and role modeling of the dolphin parent. In the end, you and your children will be closer to health, happiness, and lasting success. How can I say this with such certainty? Because we humans are hardwired to have lives of vitality and joy. It's what we're meant to achieve, so long as we work with our nature and not against it.

Prescriptions

In my office every day, I not only give prescriptions for medication but also guidance for the essentials of life. If you can believe it, I write out on a prescription pad lifestyle recommendations such as, "sleep," "eat healthy," "exercise," and "get fresh air." I also write down motivation and relationship (parenting) strategies such as "empathize," "be optimistic," "reinforce process not product," and "follow a balanced lifestyle." These prescriptions may seem overly simple, but they work incredibly well! Just like deadlines help people get projects in on time, prescriptions to sleep, play, and exercise remind my patients that they need to both pay attention to and take care of their minds, bodies, and lifestyles. If you don't sleep enough or play enough, I suggest you do so too. Writing such tasks down and thinking about them like prescriptions can keep you on track and focused. Some prescriptions are straightforward directions, some are powerful or challenging questions, and some come in a three-part form: (1) provide a favorable environment, (2) role model the behavior for your child, and (3) guide your child to act on the prescription for success. Sometimes, a favorable environment is all you need.

These prescriptions are not just for your child, by the way. They're for you as well. Integrating balance in your own life is the most powerful way to guide and role model balance for your child (plus, it's really hard to parent effectively if you're off balance).

My first set of prescriptions is for you, the parent:

- *Identify Mother Nature's signals.* How does your biology let you know that you're off balance? Some people may feel sleepy, others can't sleep, some feel irritated, others apathetic, some are affected by all of the above. What are *your* signals?
- *Identify what lifestyles illnesses you may be vulnerable to.* If you consistently ignore Mother Nature's signals, what illnesses might develop? Some may be susceptible to physical illnesses, others mental illnesses, and others both. Hint: we are often prone to illnesses that run in our genes—think of your blood relatives.
- *Identify which basic survival activities you may be doing too little of or not at all.* For example, think about how much you sleep, how much healthy food you eat, and how much exercise you get.

That's it for now! Throughout the rest of this book, you'll find prescriptions for how to implement balance in your already busy life. OK, ready? Let's dive into action!

PART 3

· ·

Taking Action:

Achieving Twenty-First-Century
Success Through Balance

Chapter 5

· · · · · · · · · · · · ·

THE BASICS ARE FIRST
AND FOREMOST

Steve was my patient and a banker who made a lot of money. But was Steve "successful"? He was putting in eighteen-hour workdays and hardly saw his children, although he felt that he "provided" for them well. Steve slept four to six hours a night and refueled on coffee, diet cola, and alcohol. His diet was terrible. He sat at a desk all day, rarely exercised, and was gaining weight. Steve recognized that he was unhealthy, but he did nothing about it. His work took priority over everything else. Steve eventually developed insomnia. His cholesterol and blood sugar levels grew. He was having severe lower back pain from sitting so much. After months of sleeplessness, pain, stress, and anxiety, his performance at work was slipping. Steve began using OxyContin to get through his day. One day, while away on business travel, Steve was found dead in his hotel room. His toxicology report showed so much alcohol and OxyContin in his blood that the coroner couldn't conclude whether Steve's overdose had been intentional or accidental.

It's easy to see where Steve went wrong now that he's dead. And yet, many of us make exactly the same mistakes Steve did every day. We live in a toxic culture where we have to work hard to maintain the basics of life. Our food is tainted, our air is bad, we sit long hours on terrible chairs, and sleep deprivation is the rule rather than the exception. Why do we live such unhealthy lives and role model such nonsense to our kids? I believe part of it is that while we can easily see what disease and illness look like, we have only a very vague sense of what it means to be healthy. We often don't know what health is until it's gone. We don't feel it slipping away from us until the symptoms of disease settle in. Health has "no symptoms." And when we're distracted, we're most at risk of losing it. We have many words for different symptoms and diseases, but very few words for health and well-being. I believe the best way to define health—whether physical, mental, social, or spiritual—is balance. And it is balance that brings vitality because health is far more than just the absence of disease.

Dolphins, like all animals, are concerned with survival first. The strange thing about humans is that despite our sophistication, we often mindlessly value our survival after much less important things, such as getting homework done instead of getting out to exercise or shopping online into the wee hours of the night instead of sleeping. Our warped priorities profoundly affect our natural and healthy feedback loops. In order to right our ships, we need to reexamine and understand the very basics of survival, and put these basics back on the top of our priorities list.

The basics are essential for adults, but they're even more so for children whose brains and bodies are developing. For children to grow up balanced, they must grow up in a balanced environment. In fact, the well-known fundamentals of neuroplasticity (the ability for the brain to adapt in form and function) *require* these basics: sleep, nutrition, exercise, and what I will call "mindfulness"—the ability to pay close attention to the world around you. That's what this chapter is about: the most neglected human needs.

You don't have to be a doctor to know that the prescriptions below are good for you. And you don't have to be sick to follow them. These are behaviors that all humans are meant to follow. But before we get deeper into the ideas of the dolphin way, let's troubleshoot the easy stuff. Just like the IT guy at work who asks you whether your computer is turned on before he starts answering your questions about why the thing isn't working properly, let's make sure we're taking care of the most basic human needs and then start solving tougher problems.

Moving towards a way of life that is healthy, happy, and truly successful requires at least two processes: (1) shaking off the unhealthy, imbalanced tiger and (2) adding in some dolphin (or balanced) behaviors. Shaking off the tiger may be all you need because health and balance are innate to a human life. Unfortunately, despite our desperate searching, we haven't found a magic wand that we can wave to get healthy. The path to health takes more effort. As Yoda said: "You have to unlearn what you have learned" and "Try not. Do ... or do not. There is no try."

PRESCRIPTION

Give Your Child Some Free Time

Build in some downtime for your child every day. Give yourself some free time while you're at it. Don't just hope it will happen. Make it happen. That's right, you may have to cancel some activities.

Your first response may be "that sounds fine, but my child likes all his activities or he gets bored" or "my child doesn't *seem* stressed." If you grow up in a particular environment, you'll crave that environment because it's the only one you know. Sure, your child may ask for this or that activity, but that doesn't mean she *needs* it. It may just mean that she doesn't know what to do without it. And that's not good. Even if she really does love everything she's doing, if she's not getting enough downtime, she's still probably stressed—needing constant stimulation is as much a sign of stress as meltdowns, crying spells, and anxiety attacks. Even when I don't feel stressed, my brain tells me when I'm too busy and yours probably does too. For me, I become even more absent-minded and will even forget really important things such as doctor's appointments! This may seem benign, but it's a symptom of my brain's stress, and we must understand that being or feeling "frazzled" means that our brains are just not working right. Not just our brains are under pressure when we're too busy, our bodies are too. When we're stressed, stress hormones such as cortisol and adrenalin are released in the body. In the short term, these hormones may help get us through our busy day. But when bodies and brains are swimming in cortisol and adrenalin day after day, the consequences are not long in coming. In the end, keep in mind that this decision is not your child's.

Of course, in some ways, we all want to be busy because that means we're important. Let's be honest, we love to talk about, post on Facebook, and blog about all the wonderful things we're doing. We also may judge the person who isn't "too busy" as lazy, unmotivated, or just not important enough to be invited everywhere and be part of everything. However, being too busy, exhausted, and sleep deprived are not status symbols at all—they just mean you're out of control.

PRESCRIPTION

Breathe Deeply and Be Mindful

No matter how far they travel, how much trouble they're in, or how busy they are, dolphins pay attention to their surroundings and breathe deeply. We humans also need to remember to keep breathing in and out calmly, regardless of what life throws at us.

Breathing deeply takes us out of the fear mode of fight, freeze, or flight, and allows us to experience the awareness of choice. Forget health and vitality, we can't even survive if we're driven by fear and are oblivious to our surroundings.

Deep, controlled breathing is the first and most powerful key to awareness and self-control, and this fact is confirmed time and time again in biology, in psychology, and in reality! Breathing is completely instinctive, but breathing deeply *is voluntary* and can be controlled. Deep, purposeful breaths trigger receptors in our expanded lungs that send signals to our brain that we are OK. When we breathe deeply, we shut down our autonomic system (our fight, freeze, and flight system) and move to an awareness of choice. If we breathe with shallow and out-of-control breaths, we build up CO_2, which tells our body that we're suffocating and need to fight, freeze, or flee. We then experience more anxiety, panic, or anger.

Breathing deeply when we eat, work, practice, socialize, or perform has two outcomes. First, it automatically relaxes us and we experience less anxiety and frustration. Second, it puts us in control of how we eat, work, practice, socialize, and perform. With deep, controlled breathing, the task we're struggling with will *always* be easier. It's simply biologically impossible to experience anxiety, panic, or anger if we're consistently breathing deeply.

Guiding children towards mindful, deep, controlled breathing offers them a lifelong tool for when they feel stressed, upset, anxious, worried, angry, or out of control. This tool will help them regulate their bodies and minds and help them think clearer when solving the problem before them. Despite these benefits, every day I see children and parents who don't know how or have simply forgotten to breathe deeply.

Controlled deep breaths are not always easy, especially in the face of anxiety, panic, and anger. However, like everything else in life, deep breathing gets easier the more you practice. For example, even though I've spoken about the advantages of deep breathing every day for over a decade, I still don't always do it. Although I know how important it is, I didn't experience the power of deep, controlled breathing until I prac-ticed it consistently. The key word here is *consistently*. Many people may say, "Yeah, I tried deep breathing. It just doesn't work for me." I used to think the same thing. There was no way a couple of deep breaths were going to help me through my emotions of hurt, anxiety, and anger. I'm delighted to tell you this: if you ever feel out of control due to your emotions, taking deep, controlled breaths will *always* help you regain control. Deep, controlled breathing as a means of self-control is simply built into our human biology. Although you may not believe it now, once you start practicing deep breathing, your life will improve. If you continue the practice, you'll see how you're moving closer to being in control of your life and not having your life's circumstances control you.

A great way to stay focused on maintaining deep, regular breathing is to practice "mindfulness" techniques. Mindfulness is a state of active, open attention on the present. For the purposes of this book, I will discuss mindfulness as a practice of "paying close attention," which means being aware of our internal and external environments. It's the practice of becoming (and being) connected to our external senses of seeing, hearing, tasting, smelling, and touching and our internal senses of feeling and thinking. Practicing mindfulness can be as simple as looking around you and noticing what's there, such as looking at your food and noticing what and how much you're about to eat. It can be as simple as looking into your child's eyes and noticing what you're seeing—a separate living being looking to you for love and guidance. Seeing your child's facial expression and hearing the tone of your child's voice can tell you far more than hours of conversation.

Sophisticated neuroimaging studies show that mindfulness improves brain anatomy. When we pay close attention, our brain releases something called *brain-derived neurotropic factor (BDNF)*—a key chemical needed for neuroplasticity. BDNF isn't released when we're multitasking. So, if you're not being mindful, you're missing out on these incredible benefits: stress reduction, better fear modulation, greater emotional regulation, greater focus, improved learning and working memory, greater satisfaction in relationships, improved immune functioning, morality, intuition, and cognitive flexibility. As a medical doctor, I can think of no better way to respond to lifestyle-related diseases than mindfulness.

I was initially skeptical about suggesting mindfulness practice to my teenage patients, thinking they would automatically reject it as something "weird." To my pleasant surprise, as I described mindfulness and its associated benefits, many of my teenage patients became interested. In some ways, children and teenagers are far more in touch with their intuition than many adults (who tend to be much more skeptical and inflexible). Some of my teenage patients have enrolled in meditation, mindfulness, or yoga classes; asked their coaches or instructors to incorporate a mindfulness activity into the first five minutes of sports practice; downloaded guided mindfulness videos; and signed up for mindfulness email and Facebook alerts. Many have simply chosen to "unplug" for a few minutes a day and try to relax. That means putting away all their devices and shutting off all their hurried thoughts for just a few minutes a day, and focusing on breathing.

Many parents have told me, "That will never happen with my child." But time and time again, it *has* happened. Whatever form of mindfulness practice children tried, those who stuck with it consistently seemed to receive the greatest benefits. I saw children and families become less agitated with their frenzied schedules or, better yet, realize their schedules were frenzied and make wise choices to cut back. I saw anxiety go down and mood go up. I saw improvements in sleep, focus, concentration, and performance; an increase in creativity; and, most of all, better connection with oneself, others, and the world. The reason for all these benefits is that mindfulness takes us off autopilot and makes us more fully alive and aware. The easiest way to be mindful is to simply breathe deeply.

Create a Favorable Environment

When our bodies and minds are relaxed, we naturally become more mindful of our internal and external states and take deeper breaths with more control. Surround your child with places and things that are known to be relaxing, such as fresh air, nature, and pets. Most children are drawn to things that naturally relax them, so sometimes all you need to do is get out of the way and let them relax.

Be a Role Model

Show your child that you value mindfulness, and deep and controlled breathing. Practice slowing down or breathing deeply a few times per day: at breakfast, in the car, during a walk, sitting at your desk, lying in your bed, or in a lineup at the coffee shop. When you're stressed or angry, try taking deep, controlled breaths right in front of your children. Even have your child help you do it. If your child sees you making the effort to do it, even though it's really hard (and you may give up too early and panic and get angry anyway), he will value it and also make an effort to do it. Keep in mind that when we operate in a stressed state, we find it harder to control our breathing, and that's all the more reason to do it.

Guide Your Child to Success

Explain the benefits of deep breathing and the drawbacks of shallow breathing to your child. For example, deep breaths signal to the brain that we're OK, and shallow breaths signal to the brain that we're in trouble. Point out real-life drawbacks of shallow breathing when they occur. If your child appears anxious or angry, ask her to notice her breathing pattern (with kindness and empathy, of course!). Show her how to take control of herself through her breathing pattern. You can also breathe deeply with her. Becoming in tune with your breathing may not be easy at first, and it may require practice. Help your child with deep breathing in a consistent way until it becomes easy for him or her.

Mindfulness Exercises

The following simple exercises can help develop mindfulness. Try four or five rounds of these exercises, and notice how your body and mind relax.

- **Balanced breathing.** Inhale for a count of four, then exhale for a count of four—all through the nose, which adds a natural resistance to the breath. You can increase your goal for six to eight counts per breath with the same objective in mind: to reduce stress by calming the nervous system and increasing focus. The key is to breathe deeply and slowly (count one-one thousand, two-one thousand, etc.). Your child can practice this anytime, anyplace—and this exercise is especially effective before bed, when racing thoughts or anxiety are distracting your child from sleep.

- **Box breathing.** Have your child slowly "draw" the shape of a box with a finger while breathing deeply. Inhale on the left upward line, hold the breath as you "draw" the top line, exhale on the right downward line, and then hold the out breath as you "draw" the bottom line. This exercise allows for a purposeful pause between inhales and exhales. Try this one before an exam, a performance, or any stressful event. You can add in a neuroplasticity "walk" in the form of a mantra or statement as well. The statement must be real to validate the anxiety but also optimistic. For example, say, "this feels scary right now" on the way up the box, pause, then say, "but it shall pass" on the way down the box, and then pause again. Try it, you'll be amazed!

PRESCRIPTION

Drink Water

Dolphins obtain the water they need from the food they eat as well as the metabolic breakdown of food (the fat-burning process releases water). Despite the life-sustaining importance of water, we humans often overlook it, and many of us are walking around dehydrated. In fact, two out of three of us don't drink enough water.[1] Coffee, tea, cola, alcohol, and flavored drinks can't take the place of water. In fact, caffeinated and alcoholic drinks are diuretics—that is, they make us pee and *rob* us of water.

Our bodies use between two and three quarts of water per day for such important functions as regulating body temperature, metabolizing nutrients, and cushioning joints, organs, and tissues. Proper hydration signals to our brains that we're OK and thus able to pursue other survival activities. It reduces irritability, fatigue, mental dullness, and anxiety. Dehydration, on the other hand, can lead to weakness, dizziness, mental confusion, mental dullness, heart palpitations, physical sluggishness, and fainting episodes.

So, why aren't we drinking enough water? Some of us simply forget, some of us were never taught to drink water over other beverages, and some are actively staying away from water to look thinner. A patient of mine passed out from dehydration after a ballet audition. When I asked why she hadn't had any water and if her parents knew about her hydration habits, she said, "Of course! I got the idea to stop drinking water before auditions from my mom. She does it all the time before she wants to fit into a new dress."

Caffeine use by young people is a growing problem. The demand for caffeine is clearly huge—just look around at all the coffee shops! Young people are drinking coffee earlier in life and also using energy drinks with high amounts of caffeine more and more. Avoid caffeine if you can. (I'm still working on that.) If you do use caffeine, limit the amount: one six-ounce beverage a day, and don't drink it past 3 P.M. at the latest.

Hydration is important. You can't parent properly and your child can't respond in a balanced and calm manner if you're both dehydrated. So, fetch your water bottles and fill them up!

Create a Favorable Environment

Try ditching all sugary drinks (including juice boxes) from your home. When I did this, my children whined for one week and then never mentioned them again.

Provide a stool or step in front of your sink if your child can't reach the tap. If the water in your area isn't safe to drink, have plenty of filtered water or water bottles available in your home. Have your child bring his or her own water bottle to school and extracurricular activities.

Be a Role Model

Drink water yourself, and drink it in front of your child. You need eight, eight-ounce glasses per day. If you're in tune with your instincts, you won't need to measure. Just drink water when you're hungry between meals, tired, or thirsty.

Guide Your Child to Success

Explain the benefits of drinking water and the drawbacks of not drinking water to your child. Connect the drawbacks with times your child didn't drink enough water (for example, maybe he was irritable because of dehydration) and the benefits with times your child did drink enough water (for example, maybe she felt more energetic after drinking water). If your child is tired, ask whether he could be dehydrated and give him water. If your child looks vibrant and energetic, ask her if she drank water that day. Explain that sugary drinks cause dehydration and that water is all you need. Ask your child to pay attention to thirst and how it can be confused for hunger.

Finally, I have a gross-sounding but very effective way to teach your children about hydration. I'm half proud and half embarrassed to say that I taught my children "the science of pee." They now understand that dark urine means they need to drink more water and that the goal is clear yellow urine. They monitor and compare their urine colors, and it's actually a fabulous way for them to see "balance" (in this case, metabolic balance) in action. It gets a bit grosser when you add in the smell analysis, so let's just leave it at that!

PRESCRIPTION

Eat Healthy

Dolphins and other animals in nature rarely, if ever, become overweight. We almost never see obesity in the wild. Mother Nature created a near-perfect regulation of our biological processes for nourishment. However, too many of us aren't eating healthy, and it's killing us. When we eat healthy foods, our bodies signal to our brains that we're OK and can pursue other activities. When we don't eat healthy and balanced foods, our bodies and brains become dysregulated and Mother Nature sends us warning signals such as hunger, fatigue, and irritability. If we consistently ignore these signals, we can become off balance and ill.

Worldwide obesity has more than doubled since 1980, and it's not just a North American problem anymore.[2] Weight-related diseases like hypertension and diabetes are on the rise worldwide. One in three adults has high blood pressure, which leads to all kinds of problems, including deadly heart disease.[3] By 2015, it's predicted that 75 percent of Americans will be overweight and 44 percent will be obese. Currently, almost two-thirds of Americans are overweight.[4] It's hard to believe, but it has now been confirmed that being over-weight is currently killing three times more people than malnutrition in human populations (with the exception of sub-Saharan Africa).[5] While obesity rates are lower in children than adults right now, they're rising fast everywhere.

Obesity is associated with a wide range of diseases. These include coronary heart disease; type 2 diabetes; cancer (endometrial, breast, and colon); hypertension (high blood pressure); dyslipidemia (high total cholesterol or high levels of triglycerides); stroke; liver and gallbladder disease; sleep apnea and respiratory problems; osteoarthritis; gynecological problems (abnormal menses, infertility); and anxiety and depression.

Cases of anorexia and bulimia have also risen, as well as partial-syndrome eating disorders, which are characterized by some symptoms of an eating disorder. Wrestlers, gymnasts, models, and performers such as dancers, singers, and actors are more at risk for these eating disorders. Eating disorders affect up to twenty-four-million Americans and seventy-million individuals worldwide.[6] Of those who have eating disorders, 90 percent are women between the ages of twelve and twenty-five.[7] Of the women surveyed on a college campus, 91 percent had attempted to control their weight through dieting, and 22 percent dieted "often" or "always."[8] While women are more commonly affected by eating disorders, more than one-million men and boys battle the illness every day.[9]

Both anorexia and bulimia are about control, but in different ways. Bulimia is characterized by out-of-control eating with cycles of binging and purging. Anorexia is often driven by overcontrol of one's body by individuals who may feel (or have felt) out of control in their lives. For example, one of the most out-of-control experiences imaginable, child-hood sexual abuse, is a strong risk factor for all the eating disorders (and many psychiatric disorders). Perfectionistic parents (that is, tiger parents) are another risk factor.

It's truly a world out of balance when it comes to our relationship with food. We've created a world where too many of us are on opposite ends of the bell curve. At the rate we're going, we're not going to have a bell curve soon. It's our parental responsibility to draw back the reins and teach our children to have a healthy relationship with food.

Create a Favorable Environment

Minimize or eliminate junk food in the house. Buy fruits, vegetables, legumes, and whole grains, and make family meals with them whenever you can. Eat for nourishment with a side benefit of social bonding—that's what dolphins do.

Create a routine of three meals and three snacks a day at regular intervals. Try to have at least one meal together as a family. Eating together as a family is a powerful predictor of future health and success. According to a number of studies, children who eat at least five times a week with their family are at lower risk of developing poor eating habits, weight problems, or alcohol and substance dependencies. They also tend to perform better academically than peers who frequently eat alone or away from home.

Be a Role Model

Show your child how much you value the importance of a balanced diet with the four food groups (whole foods) at regular intervals. Make healthy food choices in front of your children. Feel free to even tell them that you would really love a cookie or a bag of chips, but you're going to eat an apple or a banana instead. If they see you trying to eat healthy most of the time, even though you may get sidetracked, they'll understand the value you place on a balanced diet.

At meal time, sit down at the table, shut off all your devices, look at your food, eat slowly and with purpose, and comment on the taste and appearance of your food. Make eating social and fun, not work or a mindless activity.

Finally, ask yourself whether you equate body image and size with self-worth (answer honestly and bravely). If the answer is yes, seek to change this in yourself. I once heard a mother say that her daughter didn't like her dance instructor because she was "too heavy." Her daughter didn't care one bit how heavy her dance instructor was, but her mother did. By saying so right in front of her child, she planted the seed in her daughter's mind that it's OK to associate size and shape with a person's worth. Value body size and shape, but don't overvalue them. If you do, work to establish a balanced sense of a body image for yourself, and get help if you need it. If you have a healthy relationship with food, eating, body size, and body shape, chances are that your child will too.

Guide Your Child to Success

Share with your child the benefits of a healthy diet and the risks of an unhealthy diet. Explain which foods are low calorie and nutrient rich, such as fruits, vegetables, and whole grains.

Most people can still enjoy small amounts of high-fat, high-sugar, high-calorie foods as an infrequent treat. Just be sure to choose foods that promote a healthy weight and good health more often than you choose foods that don't. Identify situations that might trigger unhealthy eating, such as eating in front of the television or going to a movie and mindlessly inhaling popcorn and candies.

PRESCRIPTION

Be Active

Dolphins, like all animals, are active. Dolphins occasionally leap above the water's surface and sometimes perform acrobatic moves. Scientists aren't certain about the purpose(s) of the acrobatics. Possibilities include locating schools of fish by looking at above-water signs such as feeding birds, communicating with other dolphins, dislodging parasites, or simply having fun. Regardless of the reason, unlike humans, dolphins don't have sedentary lives. Sedentary lives and weight gain go hand in hand. Children and adults need to move.

For most of human history, we have been moving in nature, not sitting at a desk. Movement also releases BDNF. Cardiovascular exercise—any form of running around that elevates the baseline heart rate—is as effective as antidepressants for mild symptoms of depression and anxiety. Thirty to sixty minutes of exercise three times a week is beneficial in treating these conditions.[10] Exercise also improves the effectiveness of studying and test scores, possibly due to greater activation of the neurons involved in learning and long-term memory. Whether it's the increased blood flow to the brain, the release of natural dopamine, serotonin, and endorphins to improve mood and enhance attention and memory, or more likely all of the above, there's no substitute for regular movement.

But here's the thing: exercise during competitive sports isn't enough for good health; children also need recreational exercise (such as walking, running, hiking, and biking). Many of my patients get a lot of exercise in their sports leagues, but still have anxiety and depression. Why? The psychological benefits of exercise decrease when exercise is coupled with pressure, stress, and overcompetition. When children know that their coaches and parents are evaluating them and that the purpose is to win or "get better" instead of get a workout, blow off steam, or have fun, they don't experience the same mood-enhancing effects that recreational exercise offers. Dolphin parents need to ensure that their children get exercise that supports recreation. The word *recreation* is based on the prefix "re" (anew) and the root "create." It's through recreational exercise, not ultracompetitive exercise, that we become *re*charged and *re*created.

Create a Favorable Environment

Parents today have to work harder to create a favorable environment for physical activity. Modern-day staples like the car, elevator, escalator, and especially "screen time" lead to fewer opportunities to get active. Regardless, creating a lifestyle where regular outdoor and indoor activities are important isn't impossible, especially with young children who naturally run around every opportunity they get. Ensure that simple things like yard work and helping around the house are whole family tasks. An active pet such as a dog will force you outside. Take up outdoor hobbies, such as hiking, biking, swimming, camping—whatever you enjoy. Most important in today's world, limit screen time.

Limiting Screen Time

If you want your child to experience as much physical activity as possible, you have no choice but to limit screen time. When I talk to parents about exercise, one of the most common statements I hear is, "My children won't move—they just want to watch TV, surf the Net, and play video games." But these desires have to do with the environment children are in, not children's natural desire to be inactive. Young children in particular would have no access to screen time if adults didn't give it to them.

Young people spend an average of seven hours and thirty-eight minutes a day consuming "entertainment media."[11] The average American youth spends 900 hours in school each year, but watches 1,500 hours of television.

Excessive television viewing during childhood and adolescence is associated with all kinds of negative outcomes. One study showed that early exposure to television can lead to attention problems later on. The number of hours spent watching television during childhood is also associated with symptoms of attention problems in adolescence. The results remained significant after controlling for gender, attention problems in early childhood, cognitive ability at five years of age, and socioeconomic status. The results were also independent of adolescent television viewing.[12]

In addition, the effects of having a television on in the background are more subtle, but profoundly important—they include disrupting children's play. In one study, twelve- to thirty-six-month-old children who played with toys while their parents were in the same room and watching adult programs played for a shorter period of time than when the television was off. In addition, children used a less-sophisticated form of play when background television was present compared with when it wasn't.[13] It seems that the television program, even though it was mostly incomprehensible and probably boring to the children, was captivating enough to repeatedly attract their attention and distract them from playing. Not surprisingly, adults talk less to their children when the television is on—disrupting important child–parent communication.

We can't control what's on television or how violent video games are, but we can choose what we buy and control screen time. In all, 67 percent of American households play video games. About one-third of families with young children leave the television on all or most of the time.[14] The number of televisions per average American household is increasing, with 2.86 per house in 2009 to 2.93 in 2010.[15] In 2010, 55 percent of American homes had three or more televisions, and currently there are more televisions per home than there are people![16] Televisions and computers now appear in almost every room of people's homes, including bathrooms and children's bedrooms.

Like many parents, I've used screen time as a babysitter, as an incentive to do homework, as a distraction when I was trying to feed my little ones (my children were the pickiest eaters around!) and, of course, to get some peace and quiet. So, if I did all that, how can I blame my children for wanting to watch television when they're bored, for a reward, or just to relax?

Let's be honest and admit that we *are* actually in control of our homes, no matter how much our children may yell, scream, and bully. We have options: (1) the easy option: let your children do what they want with television and other screens; (2) the highly effective option: have no screens in your home at all because children get enough of them elsewhere (simple, but definitely not easy); and (3) the in-between option (which is what I've chosen for now): establish clear limits to screen time and stick to these limits under all circumstances. If you pick option two or three, please explain to your children with genuine empathy and kindness why you made this decision. Say some-thing like, "When I was a child, I used to love watching TV, so I know this is hard for you. It's not a punishment. All people need balance to stay healthy, and the amount of time you're watching TV is out of balance with the rest of the important things in life. These are the limits until we reestablish balance again ..."

Of course, children will try everything to push you to the breaking point to give up on your limits, but once they're clear that "no means no," they'll stop. The whole transition of taking back control over your home environment can take about a week—maybe less, maybe more, depending on your children and especially on how well you're able to stick to your own rules. Be prepared for a few rocky days, and please don't book something like an important dinner party during the adjustment period because your children will see the opportunity to push your limits as soon as they sense your stress. Know that if you stick to your inner dolphin, there will be less stress in your life than there was before.

Be a Role Model

Show your child that movement, activity, stretching, and exercise are important to you. If you don't take care of your body, it's likely that your child won't either. Build in activities when you can. Keep it simple. Exercise doesn't mean you have to enroll in all kinds of scheduled classes or go to the gym—although, if that works for you without added stress, that's great! However, for all of human history (until recently), humans got all the exercise they needed from being active in their daily environments. Even our parents' generation was more active; our parents didn't need to schedule in exercise as much because they simply walked a lot more. I've made a few simple choices to be more active. I walk rather than drive to places when possible and find a parking spot that's farther away from where I'm going (which makes it easier to park my minivan anyway). I take the stairs instead of the elevator. I get up from my computer every hour and stretch out my back. I tell my children how awful it feels to be sitting all day. I've started taking my children to some of my health care appointments. Just seeing me face down getting my back adjusted by my chiropractor or having needles stuck into me by my acupuncturist has given them powerful visuals of what happens to me because I didn't take care of my body earlier on. I recently started taking my oldest to yoga classes with me, and it's fantastic to be moving, stretching, breathing, and practicing mindfulness with your child right beside you.

Guide Your Child to Success

Consistent messaging, role modeling, and a favorable environment are the cornerstones of guiding your children to be more active. The most powerful way to encourage activity is to explain in a non-judgmental, kind, and empathic way why you would like them to do so—the benefits to them of being active and the drawbacks to them of not being active. Be firm, loving, and consistent—it's worth it.

PRESCRIPTION

Sleep Restfully

How do dolphins make time to sleep? Since they're mammals, sleep is a must. On the other hand, sleep could also mean drowning or falling prey to a shark. So how do dolphins manage to both sleep and stay alive? Amazingly, they sleep with only half their brain and, literally, with one eye open! One hemisphere of the dolphin brain stays active so the other half can sleep. In this way, the dolphin can go to the surface for air, stay afloat, and also look out for predators. By alternating the sides of the brain that sleep, dolphins manage to sleep for about eight hours every day. Given what dolphins have to worry about, and given the fact that they manage to sleep soundly and for long periods, we really have no excuse for being sleep deprived.

In over ten years of practice, the single most effective thing I ever do as a doctor is emphasize the healing and life-sustaining power of sleep. I've spoken to hundreds, if not thousands, of people about the importance of sleep. And I've prevented dozens of psychiatric hospitalizations simply by guiding my patients to better sleep.

Optimal brain functioning requires organization and stabilization of the neurons and corresponding structures. Sleep and dreams (REM sleep) appear to serve this purpose. Research shows that both sleep and dreams will improve memory and help bring stability to neural processes.[17] REM sleep in particular may contribute to the testing and strengthening of brain circuits and is not surprisingly most frequent during periods of brain development such as childhood and adolescence.

A Harvard Medical School study had students think of a problem they were trying to solve before going to sleep and found that a significant number of students had come up with novel solutions in their dreams![18] In a German study, participants at the University of Lübeck were shown how to solve a long, tedious math problem.[19] They were then sent for an eight-hour break during which some slept and some didn't. Upon retesting, those who had slept during the break were more than twice as likely to figure out a simpler way to solve the problem than those who had not slept. Of course, we don't need a study to know that we all function better after having a good night's sleep.

The feeling of well-being that comes from having had enough sleep is a signal for us to do it again. But we seem to have forgotten that we have a biological need for sleep. Unfortunately, exhaustion and sleep deprivation have become a kind of bizarre status symbol for some. When we don't sleep restfully, Mother Nature sends us warning signals and flashing lights such as fatigue, poor concentration, and anxiety. If we don't heed those warnings, our bodies become dysregulated, and we can no longer sleep (that is, we can experience insomnia) even if we have the time to do so.

In the human body, sleep basically regulates ... well, everything. Sleep deprivation leads to a variety of short- and long-term problems, such as the following:

- **Hormonal changes that can lead to weight gain.** Sleep deprivation has been linked to the dysregulation of ghrelin—the hormone that stimulates appetite and increases insulin, and is partly responsible for turning food into fat.[20]
- **Decreased performance and alertness.** We tell people to "get a good night's sleep" before a big event for a good reason. One night of poor sleep, with only a ninety-minute reduction in sleep time, is associated with up to 33 percent impairment in daytime alertness.[21]
- **Memory and cognitive impairment.** After twenty-four hours of sleep deprivation, response times for tasks testing memory maintenance and manipulation were significantly slower than after a typical night's rest.[22]
- **Poor quality of life.** Sleep deprivation can lead to long-term problems such as high blood pressure, heart attack, heart failure, stroke, obesity, psychiatric problems (including depression and

other mood disorders), attention deficit disorder (ADD), mental impairment, fetal and childhood growth retardation, and insomnia.[23]

Students who don't sleep enough are at a serious disadvantage. Sleep has extensive effects when it comes to schoolwork. In one study, students who got As and Bs were found to go to bed forty minutes earlier and get around twenty-five minutes more sleep than those students who were struggling and failing.[24] In addition, the longer the students stayed up on weekends, the worse their grades. This study also examined the behavior, moods, and feelings during the day based on "adequate" or "less than adequate" sleep patterns. Students who slept less than six hours and forty-five minutes per night and students who slept in more than two hours later than their peers had daytime sleepiness, sleep/wake behavior problems, and depressive moods.

The good news for those with insomnia and other disorders related to sleep deprivation is that with education and treatment, memory and cognitive deficits improve and the number of related injuries and other health problems decrease.

I used to be surprised at how stunned people were when I advised them of this basic biological need. I once found myself telling a cardiologist that his wife, who was suffering from severe post-partum depression, really just needed some sleep. He wanted to fly her to the Mayo Clinic for a "full workup," including a CT scan and MRI of her brain. I assessed her and discovered that she hadn't slept more than four hours in a row for over four months. That kind of sleep deprivation will cause you to lose touch with reality. I asked the cardiologist to wait a few days before he took his wife across the continent and away from their three children. After four days of solid sleep, although she was still depressed and in need of treatment, she was no longer confused and experiencing psychosis. Now, you would think a cardiologist would know the survival value of sleep, but that's how far astray we are as a society—even I myself need a reminder at times!

Young people are often sleep deprived. The Centers for Disease Control recommend that children from the ages of ten through seventeen sleep at least eight-and-a-half to nine-and-a-half hours a night.[25]

Elementary school children need eleven hours of sleep a night and high school students need around nine to ten hours. Anything less constitutes sleep deprivation.

Without enough sleep, our minds are neither rested nor alert. And when we're tired and sleep deprived, we're least likely to be creative, spontaneous, caring, respectful, responsible, independent, and interested in problem solving.

Create a Favorable Environment

A routine that's strong yet flexible will help create a favorable environment for restful sleep. Try to get your child to go to bed at roughly the same time every night and wake up at about the same time every morning. However, be flexible. Humans run on a twenty-five-hour rhythm, and when each of us needs rest can vary slightly. For example, if your child is a napper, let her nap (just not more than two hours and not later than six hours before bedtime). If your child is a night owl, let him stay up later on weekends as along as his sleep remains regulated.

Be a Role Model

Establish a healthy sleep routine and environment in your own life. And, yes, that means saying no to a lot of things that keep you busy.

A common cause of sleep deprivation among the many postpartum women I've worked with is not their babies but all the things they "have to do." The visitors, thank-you cards, Facebook posts, cleaning, and "image control" all take up precious time for sleep. Postpartum is a time in which we're in survival mode; and it's a time in which we must let go of perfection. The "Oh my God, you don't even look like you had a baby" comment is not necessarily a good thing. You did just have a baby. Why are you trying to hide it? It's OK for you and your house to look like "you just had a baby," so get some sleep!

As your children get older, if you're tired, let them know it's because you didn't sleep well. The days you sleep well, let them know how good you feel. Don't walk around like a sleep-deprived zombie or they'll think that's normal and will follow suit.

Guide Your Child to Success

Explain the benefits of restful sleep and the drawbacks of poor sleep to your child. Connect real-life benefits with good sleep—maybe they had a great day or did well at something that's important to them after a lot of rest. Connect real-life drawbacks with sleep deprivation—like a meltdown, poor performance, or poor social interaction.

Remove all televisions, computers, and other electronic devices from the bedroom. This one is non-negotiable. Having screens in the bedroom sets up lifelong poor sleep habits. In addition, the white lights from screens can overstimulate our retinas and delay the release of melatonin, which we need to sleep well. Some new devices will be using blue light to mitigate this effect, but blue light is not the solution. Keeping screens out of the bedroom is.

When it comes to sleep, I can be an orca. Our home simply doesn't function well if even one of us is sleep deprived. I have clear rules and consequences for missing sleep—for myself, my children, my husband, our gecko (everyone!). I have also spent *a lot* of time explaining the importance of sleep to my children. I even have a model of the brain in each of their rooms. When it comes to sleep, I can definitely be imposing—but always collaborative. Just the other day, I said the following to my children at bedtime (Why do they always have so much fun, and look so cute, just before bed?): "I can tell you children are having a blast, but if you EVER want to have another sleepover with your friends, you need to show me you really understand how important sleep is. I know you understand this and will go to bed quickly."

A Note about Teenagers and Sleep Sleep rhythms seem to shift during adolescence. Perhaps, initially, this shift occurred to prepare teenagers for the transition into adulthood where they needed to be comfortable in the darkness of night to hunt, gather, and stay safe. For whatever reason, the teenage sleep shift is real, and teenagers have a hard time getting to sleep at 9 P.M. or even 10 P.M. Negotiate a reasonable bedtime with them—most teenagers will say 11 P.M. or 12 P.M. Then work with them to stick with it. If this bedtime doesn't allow for the nine to ten hours they need, then find out where they can make up for it—such as a nap during the day.

If your teenager is dead to the world in the mornings, ask her to see whether she can organize a first period spare so that she can sleep in. If that's not possible, ask her to see whether she can arrange to have her first class on a subject she enjoys (Who would be motivated to get out of a deep slumber to go to a class they dislike?). Encourage a nap after school, but for no more than one hour and no closer to six hours before bedtime. Let teenagers sleep in on the weekends, and, yes, that may mean until noon. If they're in a deep sleep, their bodies and minds likely need it.

Now That We Know How to Survive, How Can We Thrive?

So breathing deeply, being mindful, drinking water, eating healthy, being active, and sleeping restfully are all essential for our very survival—that's why nature has hardwired positive and negative feedback loops for these survival activities into our biology. When we do these activities in a balanced way, we can survive. However, aren't we meant to experience more than just surviving? The answer unequivocally is yes. We're meant to thrive and experience a life of vitality and joy. Not only can our children achieve vitality and joy, but we can too. We just need to listen to the clues Mother Nature gives us. Now, let's go through the other activities we're heavily rewarded for. Get ready for your light to shine brightly as you find your inner dolphin!

Chapter 6

PLAY IS IN OUR NATURE

In the 1920s, British anthropologist Gregory Bateson traveled to Papua New Guinea to study the Baining people, an indigenous group. After living among the Baining for fourteen months, he had become "bored" and frustrated with his project. Bateson found the Baining culture to be very mundane, with few myths, stories, festivals, religious traditions, or puberty rites. The activities the Baining did do were highly structured; for example, their dances were made up of rigid rules that were to be followed precisely. Bateson finally left Papua New Guinea in frustration. He stated that the Baining were "unstudiable" because of their inability to say anything interesting about their lives. He also noted "their failure to exhibit much activity beyond the mundane routines of daily work, and ... that they lived 'a drab and colorless existence.'"[1]

Bateson was not the only anthropologist to reach this conclusion. Forty years later, Jeremy Pool, a graduate student in anthropology, said the same thing after living among the Baining for a year. Apparently, the experience led Pool to leave his doctoral dissertation in anthropology and pursue computer science!

Both Bateson and Pool—people who were interested and trained to study cultures—left their study projects with the Baining people in exasperation, concluding that the Baining are so boring that there's really nothing about them of interest to observe. However, another anthropologist, Jane Fajans, was able to learn something about the Baining that has wider implications about the effects on a culture when play is devalued.[2] Fajans discovered that the Baining associate play and "childish" behavior with the behavior of animals. They believe that humans should not and must not display any behaviors that resemble play and thus, they do everything they can to discourage it in children and in adults. Their "very mundane culture" and "drab and colorless existence" was concluded to be directly due to this lack of play.

I can relate to the feelings of frustration these anthropologists experienced with what they considered to be a dull and mundane people. It's not that far from my own experiences with young people from extreme tiger families. I've always prided myself on being able to "talk to anyone about anything," but I've found it difficult to maintain interactions with extreme tiger youth because the flow of communication is so constricted. Stuart Brown, founder of the National Institute for Play, noticed something similar in Stanford University sophomores. For twelve years, he presented a fall seminar on play to a selection of Stanford sophomores, which was followed with their participation in a two-week leadership immersion. Stuart had the following to say about these students and play:

> Something I have noticed is how consistently bright these
> students all are, but as admission to Stanford became
> more competitive in recent years, I have also noticed that

their sense of autonomy has diminished. They appeared to me, at least, to initiate less and less spontaneous joy than in years past. They seemed to be in command of more information combined with consistent radar honing them in to be *pleasing* to the professors. With a few exceptions, they are, in my opinion, suffering from chronic low-grade play deprivation, and are so used to their hectic, pressured, high-performance lives (despite still being children) that they don't realize what they have missed in the pursuit of academic excellence and success.[3]

For people of every age, play is directly linked to the development of the brain's prefrontal cortex[4]—the brain region responsible for discriminating relevant from irrelevant information, goal direction, abstract concepts, decision making, monitoring and organizing our thoughts and feelings, delaying gratification, and planning for the future. The prefrontal cortex directs our highest levels of thinking and functioning. It's the part of our brains that evolved last and also develops last in human development; its full maturation doesn't happen until our mid-twenties.

For the young of all animals, the amount of time spent playing is tied to the rate and size of growth of the cerebellum, which contains more neurons than the rest of the brain. In addition to motor control, coordination, and balance, the cerebellum is responsible for key cognitive functions such as attention and language processing. Active play stimulates brain-derived neurotropic factor, which stimulates nerve growth. It also promotes the creation of new neuron connections between areas that were previously disconnected. Our desire to play is so important to our survival that the impulse to play is just as fundamental as our impulse to sleep or eat.

Play is essential to the development of the four CQ skills (creativity, critical thinking, communication, and collaboration) we need for twenty-first-century success.

All play isn't equal, however. My son is on a soccer team and plays every week for most of the year. He wears a uniform, shin pads, and cleats, and plays on a perfectly symmetrical field with measured, carefully laid-out boundaries. The rules are clear, and the coach (or referee, during a game) enforces them. When there's a disagreement, everyone looks to the coach to solve the problem, which he does swiftly. Being part of a soccer team has been a great opportunity for my son to develop soccer skills. But because of the formalized nature of the activity, it isn't a particularly good opportunity to engage in the play that develops CQ.

Think about how playing in a structured sport differs from the following experience. One day, my sons and four other neighborhood children were playing street hockey. After a while, they got tired of the game. Some of the boys wanted to go inside, others wanted to play soccer. They talked about it, and the majority, who opted for soccer, won out. They didn't have a field, per se, so they made their own field with the hockey sticks and odds and ends in the backyard: an old bike and a lawn chair served as one goal, and two trees served as the other. They spotted a couple of problems early on: the boys were of different ages and skill levels, and the backyard was slanted, both of which would make it difficult to keep things "fair." So, they had to negotiate to keep things fair. Because the slant gave an advantage to the team on the upper end, the lower-end team got an extra player. The boys negotiated the rules and adjusted them as they went along. Once in a while, I could hear a fight break out. Knowing that they would have to stop playing if they couldn't get along, they worked things out. They even cleaned up after themselves when the game was over.

I'm not sure whether the boys improved any soccer skills, but I do know that they used bucket loads of creativity, critical thinking, communication, and collaboration.

Some of the oldest forms of play provide some of the richest experiences. Hide and seek, for example, teaches children the joy of exploration and autonomy and the joy of being wanted and found. When children first run off, they feel excited and happy to be autonomous, but over time the excitement fades and the longing to be together with others begins. The tension is built up during moments of suspense and is then released when they're found. It's at this moment they're reassured of the feelings of being wanted and loved. Hide and seek teaches them that relationships are strong and that even when we're separated from others, we'll eventually come back together.

Even play that has gone sour can be just as valuable as play that brings forth smiles and whoops of joy. Let's take the oh-so-common "that's not fair" you hear when children are playing. When children play, they get a self-guided tour on what is and what isn't fair. They also find out whom to trust and not to trust, and they learn the natural consequences of being untrustworthy or unfair themselves.

Stuart Brown tells a story about the managers at Caltech's Jet Propulsion Laboratory (JPL) that shows just how important play is to our children's future success in life.[5] The managers noticed that although the younger engineers had high grades from top universities, they lacked the problem-solving skills and creativity of the older engineers. When they tried to figure out why this was, they discovered that the older engineers played and explored more as children. They found that many of them had engaged specifically in vigorous hands-on play as children. They were the children who took apart clocks and put them back together, built soapbox racing cars, and fixed appliances. The new generation had fabulous résumés, but they had done very little of this kind of play. To make sure JPL was hiring the employees who had engaged in this kind of play, they shifted their interview process to incorporate questions about job applicants' play backgrounds, which, in turn, improved their staff's ability to tackle and resolve tough engineering design challenges. As Albert Einstein said, "Play is the highest form of research."[6]

If you want your children to be intelligent, let them play. If you want them to develop emotional regulation, let them play. If you want them to be innovative, let them play. And if you want them to be able to work in a team and have great people skills, let them play. Did you notice I did not say "tell" them to play or book a play activity, or drive them around, or pay someone to instruct them to play? If you want your children to access one of the most important and powerful predictors of intelligence and healthy development, all you have to do is stay out of the way and let them play.

Developing CQ Through Play

"The debt we owe to the play of imagination is incalculable,"[7] said Carl Jung. I couldn't agree more. Play is in our nature. All mammals take time out of their day to play, despite the stress of living in nature where a predator could eat you at any moment.

Dolphins are known to play with seaweed, with bubbles, through acrobatics, through whistles and squeaks, and even with humans. Dolphins often gravitate towards "best friends"; that is, other dolphins with similar play interests. It seems that through play, dolphins learn to interact with one another and the world around them. They use play to learn and practice all those skills they need to succeed in the vast, diverse, and often dangerous waters of the world's oceans and important rivers. Dolphin play can involve strategy, competition, and a lot of time developing hunting and fighting skills. During play, dolphins also seem to connect with one another, practice their swimming, and fine-tune their navigation skills. Play-jumping in the air, another favorite form of play, may also be practice for future navigation and hunting—or maybe it's just for fun.

Dolphins and humans are among the most playful species on our planet. In fact, a strong positive correlation exists between how much an animal plays and the relative size of their brains. Dolphins, who have the second-biggest brain size next to humans, may be overtaking us when it comes to play time.

What Is Play?

Let me clarify what I mean by play. Generally speaking, play involves two kinds of thinking: divergent and convergent. Divergent play is unstructured, free, and about exploring different ways to do something versus learning the "right way" to do something. It requires creativity because it allows for exploration; there are no absolute right answers in divergent play. Convergent play, on the other hand, is less creative because it involves structure, rules, or a "correct" answer, like some video games (not all) and, of course, modern LEGO (don't get me started again). Throughout this chapter, when I refer to *play*, I'm talking about unstructured, divergent play.

Play has numerous benefits:

- *It requires trial and error.* Play is a child's first opportunity to make mistakes and learn to take failure in stride. Mistakes and failure allow children to get back up, try again, and figure things out. Trial and error is essential to adaptability, a key ingredient in human success.

- *It allows us to discover new things.* Why do you think children and adults delight in the surprise or discovery of a new toy, a new book, a new movie, a new experience, a new friend, a new way of doing something? It's simple—the human brain releases dopamine when it learns new things, and we're rewarded with a sense of well-being or joy. The transitional brain (ages twelve to twenty-four), which is the most sensitive to dopamine, gets the biggest release—causing that age group to be known as "novelty junkies" (or what they were known as before the tiger stood in their way). So why would the human brain work in a way that makes young people want to try new things? The love of novelty pushes young people to try new things (play) and leads them to explore their world. Discovery is essential to fleeing the nest and making a life for oneself.
- *It's inherently fun.* Fun is the key to exploring one's passions and relieving stress, both of which are critical for happiness.
- *It helps develop team skills.* Play teaches children how to bond socially and helps them develop the values of trust, sharing, and fairness—which are essential for developing character and leadership.
- *It improves our ability to innovate and create.* Play includes observing, questioning, experimenting, socializing, and networking—key activities in the development of CQ.
- *It helps us deal with new challenges.* Because play allows us to imagine, communicate, problem solve, experiment, collaborate, try and fail, think outside the box, and create, it helps us develop the cognitive skills we need to survive and thrive in the twenty-first century.

Forms of Play

Play and exploration (which I'll refer to simply as *play*) help us avoid taking our lives too seriously and lead us to mindfully explore our external and internal worlds. Play is so engaging that hours pass without notice; this engagement is what athletes call "the zone" or artists call "their flow." Play is mindfulness in its most fascinating form.

The National Institute for Play describes various kinds of play, which are listed below.[8]

Play via Body Movement

As hunter-gatherers, humans experienced substantial growth in our critical-thinking and problem-solving skills. We learned to think in motion, taking in and processing vast amounts of information from the environment and generating an appropriate response.[9]

The link between movement and learning is just as strong today. By moving our bodies, we move our minds. And children who play by jumping, running, twirling, throwing, and catching are thinking in motion. Scientists at the National Institute of Play believe that "innovation, flexibility, adaptability, [and] resilience have their roots in movement."[10] They also believe that play via body movement teaches us about the world around us and prepares us for "the unexpected and unusual." To me, that sounds like thinking on your feet, and I'll never look at children playing tag the same way again!

Object Play

I knew my intuition to have my son play in the dirt was correct. As it turns out, playing in the dirt teaches us about a lot more than just dirt! By manipulating objects (for example, banging sticks together, skipping rocks, and moving sand through our fingers), we're developing complex circuits in the brain that encourage exploration, assessment of safety, and how to use the attributes of objects as tools.

Playing with different types of objects helps the brain develop more than strictly physically manipulative skills. For example, studies have found that "a deficiency in fixing things by hand during one's youth may well mean deficiencies in complex problem solving in challenging work settings as an adult."[11] For example, building models and fixing cars in high school may help a young person become a good research engineer. The connection between object manipulation in childhood and higher cognitive skills such as problem solving is the subject of the wonderful book *The Hand: How Its Use Shapes the Brain, Language, and Human Culture* by neuroscientist Frank W. Wilson.[12] In it, Wilson argues that the human brain evolved intimately in connection with the human hand, and powerful mental processes occur through freely exploring our physical environments.

Imaginative and Pretend Play

Through imaginative and pretend play, we learn the power of our own minds. Full imaginative play is highly stimulating for the brain, which makes perfect intuitive sense. Why wouldn't the brain be working its hardest when it has nothing other than itself to work with! When children engage in imaginative play, their exploration is limitless—they explore whatever ideas, roles, and scenarios their minds think of. Imaginative and pretend play are not only vital to normal development but also key to enhancing children's capacity for cognitive flexibility and creativity.[13] Studies support the idea that children who have imaginary friends in childhood have a higher IQ and greater creativity in adulthood.[14] Children with a wild imagination are comfortable with cognitive uncertainty. They're able to "make up stuff" that doesn't exist and expand their thinking beyond the unknown. Like all play, imaginary play develops important emotional and social skills. In fact, empathy can simply be defined as "imagin[ing] what it feels like to be that person."[15]

Imaginative play can be truly transformative. When we imagine fantasy-based worlds, we bend the reality of our own lives and allow creativity to lead us to new ideas. What would have happened if Einstein hadn't first imagined himself flying at the speed of light! Imagination is by far the primary ingredient for what's in demand in this rapidly changing twenty-first century. Without it, we can't innovate or adapt.

Social Play

People play with others not only because it's fun but also because they're driven by the urge to be accepted and belong. Social play is actually essential for the feeling of belonging to occur. Consider the scenario of co-workers who work together for years but never really feel connected to one another or their companies until they "play" together in activities such as company golf tournaments, recreational excursions, and social events. Social play includes attunement play, rough-and-tumble play, and celebratory or ritual play.

Attunement Play Whenever an infant first smiles at his or her parent, social play has begun. When a parent and infant lock eyes, the child (and the parent) will experience joy and excitement. The parent begins to babble and coo and smile, and so does the baby. Studies using EEG and other imaging technologies have shown that the right cerebral cortex, which controls emotions, is attuned in both the infant and parent during such interactions.[16]

Rough-and-Tumble Play Rough-and-tumble play teaches us about the limits of pushing and pulling, the balance of forward and backward motion, and social interaction. If you've ever adopted a kitten who was taken away from her littermates at too young an age, you'll notice that she'll bite too hard and fully extend her claws when playing. She does so because she never got the proper feedback from her brothers and sisters about what's too rough. Like kittens, preschool children are believed to develop emotional regulation and social awareness through pushing, pulling, wrestling, and being physically chaotic. Rough-and-tumble play has been shown "to be necessary for the development and maintenance of social awareness, cooperation, fairness and altruism."[17] In fact, the greatest impact of rough-and-tumble play is in the social domain—it's thought to help children encode and decode social signals.[18]

A lack of tension control, experienced by some children who don't play sports or games that include tension, has been proven to lead to poor control over violent impulses later in life.[19] "For boys especially, rough-and-tumble play in early childhood provides a scaffold for learning emotion-regulation skills related to managing anger and aggression."[20]

Note to moms like me: let children get physical. As long as there's no bloodshed, it is truly good for them. Plus, with all this evidence, I found myself encouraging my children, including my little girl, to play fight and wrestle! Initially, letting my husband wrestle with them was hard, but having them fight with each other was unbearable. Once I took a deep breath and let them do what came naturally to them, I saw that no matter how horrible it looked, they rarely ever hurt each other. I noticed that my children only wrestle and play fight with those they're close to—siblings, cousins, and a few close friends. I've even joined in myself sometimes, and I'm in awe of how all of us can push, pull, kick, and be rough and tumble all the while squealing with delight (now, that's a lot of dopamine!).

Celebratory or Ritual Play Celebratory or ritual play teaches us how to keep social patterns in check. Birthday parties, holiday festivities, and sports galas are all times children and adults play in celebration and ritual. I've attended a number of Indian weddings, where there's time to sing, dance, and spend time with others. These affairs can last up to a month and can include hundreds of people. While they may seem overwhelming to people from other cultures, for many they're a chance for the whole—and I mean *whole!*—family, community, and pod to play together.

Storytelling Play

Could there be anything more pervasive across human cultures than storytelling? When a child is telling stories, she's discovering and practicing one of the most powerful human tools for motivation around. In Western medicine, we're trained to eliminate storytelling in favor of science, but when it comes to motivation, storytelling is far more powerful than scientific studies—and that's why we see it used more and more in advertising! Storytelling helps us make sense of the world, understand life's lessons, and—in a magical way—never forget them! Our kids need to be able to write their own stories, rather than wait for advertisers and movie producers to write them on their behalf.

Play or Die

We feel great when we engage in play—whether we're a child playing in the waves or an adult exploring a new city. Mother Nature is so determined to have us play that when we do, she generously rewards us through doses of dopamine. Why is that the case? Why are we rewarded so much to play and explore?

Play helps with early skills development (think of young dolphins practicing to hunt through play), but play is so much more than that. When an activity is so heavily rewarded by dopamine and so pervasive across species, you know it's of utmost importance to survival. It's so important, I'm considering making T-shirts and bumper stickers that say, "Play or Die."

To explain why, let me take you to the world of rats. Researchers took two groups of rats and only allowed one group to play (which, for rats, means squeaking, wrestling, and jostling).[21] Rats who were prevented from playing couldn't process minute-to-minute social cues and were either too aggressive or too passive with one another. When researchers put something new and advantageous in front of them, they took a while to use it. When researchers put something dangerous in front of them, such as a collar that smelled like a cat, the rats retreated into a hole and never came out. That's right, they *never* came out. They died in the hole! Compare those rats to the rats who were allowed to play: they, too, went into the hole when they smelled the cat, but they then explored their environment with caution and awareness; they began to test things again and eventually ventured out of the hole and lived a full and happy rat life.

During play, young people develop the coping skills and creativity they need for adulthood. Unfortunately, a lot of children these days are similar to those rats that didn't play and died in the hole. They just don't know what to do or how to figure things out.

Many scientists believe that if it wasn't for the teenage brain's enhanced sensitivity to dopamine while engaging in new experiences, it's likely that humans wouldn't have migrated across the globe or even survived as a species. The move away from home is the most difficult developmental step a human can take—as well as the most critical. That's why the tools for successful independence—play (including exploration) and novelty (an inherent part of play)—are heavily rewarded by our biology.

Play provides us with the cognitive framework and flexible thinking needed to adapt to any situation. Adaptation isn't just a physical process of evolving into something more useful, such as the famous example of Darwin's finches' beaks. Adaptation simply means being well equipped to handle the specific conditions of a local environment. While physical adaptation takes many generations, intellectual adaptation is something we can control in the here and now—it is constant calibration. A key to that is play. One could say that play gives us the tools to "make lemons out of lemonade." This type of thinking also allows us to have a sense of humor in handling conflict and stress (recall that the mature adaptive style and humor are key contributors to long-term adult wellness, happiness, and success according to George Vaillant's Grant Study of Adult Development [see Chapter 3]).

In essence, play provides us with the cognitive skill set we all need to adapt in childhood and as adults. For decades, therapists have been using play to understand and help child patients. Indeed, the field of play therapy has proven to be an effective tool for treating childhood issues such as trauma, attention deficit hyperactivity disorder (ADHD), anxiety, and depression. The goal of play therapy is to help children resolve their problems freely and work towards solutions that are best suited for their personality. What's really amazing is how well play therapy works. You can't believe the comments children make during therapeutic play—things that they would never tell you during talk therapy, things that are often kept secret or that are buried deep in the bottom of their hearts.

We all need play, adults just as much as children. I've seen many adults over the years "who have it all." They have a comfortable life with good health, financial security, and social supports. Yet they still complain that "something is missing." When these adults reintroduce play into their lives—a music class, an interesting project at work, a dance class, a golf game, traveling, gardening, hiking, or simply exploring for fun—they experience an added sense of well-being in their lives. Play also helps us find our interests and passions.

Play Personalities

Do we all engage in play in the same way? According to Stuart Brown, we tend to play via roughly eight broad personalities: the storyteller, the artist/creator, the collector, the competitor, the director, the explorer, the joker, and the mover.[22] These "play personalities" are neither absolute nor exclusive of one another. Many people enjoy aspects of many or even all eight. Early play provides vital clues to our natural strengths and interests. When we play or grow according to these strengths and interests, we're rewarded with good feelings via a release of dopamine. Why does our biology make us feel happy when we follow our natural passions? Many people forget the second part of species survival—the first part is *survival of the fittest* (the ability to adapt) and the second part is *diversity of the species.*

We need all of these play personalities to survive as a species. In an ever-changing environment, when faced with a threat to our survival, who knows if the solution will lie in the mind of the artist/creator or the collector. For complex problems, we need the diverse play personalities to collaborate and exchange ideas for solutions. If we were all engineers, who would cure the world of the bubonic plague? If we were all doctors, who would know how to deal with a flood? If there were no storytellers, how would we pass down knowledge? And if there were no musicians, how would we bond socially? We're meant to be diverse because we require minds that think in different ways to solve the ever-changing problems we face. Play provides the feelings of well-being and joy that lead us to pursue our interests to develop that diversity. Without play, we're not diverse; without diversity, we can't adapt; without adaptation, we can't survive.

As you can see, we're hardwired to play and to find and follow our natural interests. Anyone who has ever been forced to do something they've no interest in doing knows that it's torture. One person's dream of performing on stage may be another's worst nightmare. There's a reason why some people are driven to be artists, entrepreneurs, teachers, and engineers. It's unnatural for us to be the same. It's natural for us to have a wide diversity of interests and talents. We're strong in the need to play as a means of adaptation but flexible in how we play to develop diverse interests and skill sets.

We find our passions and talents through play, often unexpectedly, and through our own drive. Our passions and talents can't be instilled in us or imposed on us by someone else, not even our parents. Parents can guide their children towards their passions and talents, but they can't find or cultivate them on their children's behalf.

I'm not saying that we're all supposed to make careers out of our play personalities. However, if you can, you're one of the lucky people who love their job enough to say it doesn't feel like work. For most of us, the reality is that we can't avoid "work." For us, trying our best to incorporate our interests into our work and other parts of our lives is at least honoring that part of our biology. By ignoring the importance of play in our lives—as children and adults—we're not being true to our nature and our biology. When we're not true to our nature and biology, we become out of balance, and we lose our vitality.

Tigers Destroy Play

The United Nations High Commissioner for Human Rights has recognized play as a fundamental right of every child. But over the last two decades, "children have lost eight hours of free, unstructured, and spontaneous play a week."[23] A variety of possible factors might explain why, including "a hurried lifestyle, changes in family structure, and increased attention to academics and enrichment activities at the expense of recess or free child-centered play."[24] Schools across the world are doing away with recess to make more time for structured academics. The amount of time children spend in organized sports has doubled. Children are spending 50 percent less time outdoors, and the amount of time spent in passive activities such as video games has increased from thirty minutes in 1997 to three hours in 2003.[25]

I would ask you to consider play deprivation as no different than sleep deprivation. Both are harmful for adults, but we can sustain them for periods of time because our brains are already developed (for the most part). For children and teenagers, sleep and play deprivation during the most rapid period of brain development can be devastating.

Let's take the huge and growing problem of ADHD. Jaak Panksepp and colleagues, who study play in rats at Bowling Green University, have shown a connection between lack of rough-and-tumble play and ADHD.[26] Play reduces the impulsivity normally seen in rats who have damage to their frontal lobes, a type of brain thought to model human ADHD. Panksepp and colleagues concluded that "'abundant access to rough-and-tumble play' reduces the inappropriate hyperplayfullness and impulsivity of rats with frontal lobe damage, ... [and] a regimen of social, boisterous play might be one way to help children with mild to moderate ADHD control impulsivity (and it is also good for those not necessarily prone to ADHD)."[27]

Based on what I've seen in over ten years of working with a number of children with ADHD, I agree with this theory in many ways. Children deprived of play (especially rough-and-tumble play) in their homes and at school often develop oppositional behaviors. They're often labeled with "conduct disorder" or "oppositional defiant disorder"; sometimes they're just described as "bad kids." Parents or schools may respond to these children's behaviors with even more play deprivation as a punishment. The result is that these children's brains are unintentionally forced to develop in an imbalanced way. Once these children become adolescents, this imbalance can turn into all kinds of maladaptive behaviors, including cutting, acting out, depression, anxiety, and substance use.

Lack of play, it turns out, can result in the most disturbing behaviors out there. In 1966, a former US Marine and University of Texas Engineering student named Charles Whitman climbed up to the top of the central tower of the University of Texas's Austin Campus and, with a trunk full of weapons, ammunition, and supplies, killed fourteen people and wounded an additional thirty-one.[28] It was later discovered that before he appeared on campus, Whitman had killed his wife and mother. These horrific events left the whole nation asking the same question: Why? After looking into Whitman's records, his motive became even less clear. Whitman had never shown any signs of violence, had no criminal record, was a former altar boy, and had been the youngest American to become an Eagle Scout.

Stuart Brown, the advocate of play I mentioned earlier, is a psychiatrist who was drawn to the subject after being a panel member on this mass murder. After looking into every detail of Whitman's life, Brown and his team came upon an interesting conclusion. They found that Whitman's father had been abusive and overbearing, completely crushing Charles' natural playfulness. Brown and his team theorized the following:

> A lifelong lack of play deprived Whitman with opportunities to view life with optimism, test alternatives, or learn the social skills that, as part of spontaneous play, prepare individuals to cope with stress. The committee concluded that lack of play was a key factor in Whitman's homicidal actions—if he had experienced regular moments of spontaneous play during his life, they believed he would have developed the skill, flexibility, and strength to cope with the stressful situations without violence.[29]

Brown began looking into other murderers in Texas. The more cases he examined, a trend began to appear: the play histories of the murderers were much different from those who grew up similarly but were able to cope and act as functioning members of society. These murderers had forms of severe play deprivation that began in childhood and persisted into adulthood.

Brown ended up compiling over 6,000 play histories of a wide range of people and found that play deprivation can lead to many consequences in the long term, such as lost productivity, reduced creativity, and mild depression.[30] Brown's studies have been supported by many others, which have also shown that the prevalence of depression, stress-related diseases, interpersonal violence, addictions, and other health and well-being problems can be linked, much like a deficiency disease, to prolonged play deprivation. Conversely, successful individuals experienced a rich play life over the course of their lives. It was also found that if play was not carried into adulthood, individuals could lose emotional, social, and cognitive skills.

Childhood play deprivation turns me into a very particular kind of dolphin: the killer whale! I feel so strongly and so passionately that this essential survival activity is under serious threat that my inner orca surfaces. I've never been more disappointed in myself than when I look back on how I handled play in my early years as a parent. Even though I knew intuitively that play was important, I still let the tiger in me stand in the way. Thankfully, because I had three children back-to-back while working full time, I was a distracted tiger and my children played a lot in spite of me. I also had my children's grandparents reminding me to "just let them play." I also naively thought all was good because, when compared with other children, my children still played a lot more. What I didn't realize at the time was that as a society, we're so far off the mark when it comes to play that even though my children were playing more than others, they were still play deprived. I wish I could turn back time or squeeze into my children's little brains and connect those neurons for them, but I can't. However, now I'm so fired up about play that if anyone tries to mess with my children's play, I go orca on them!

Luckily, Mother Nature is generous and forgiving, so it's never too late to change. Laboratory evidence shows that a play deficit may be much like a sleep deficit. Just as we can catch up on sleep, research shows that animals deprived of play will engage in rebound play when allowed to do so again.[31] Research also shows that when you bring recess back, children bounce back and behave better in school.[32] When we do finally play again, our brains feel optimistic and creative, we're more likely to embrace the new again, and we want to test and push the boundaries of our skills.[33]

So let me get out my prescription pad for more play for you and your children. Of course, the first prescription will be to regain some balance.

PRESCRIPTION

Shake Off the Overprotective Tiger

Overprotective tigers leave their children with no opportunity for exploration. By hovering and directing in sports, academics, music, and other activities, they deny children's natural tendencies to play and explore freely. Overprotection stands in the way of children becoming healthy, happy, and successful in the twenty-first century.

Shaking off the overprotective tiger simply means giving your child (and yourself) some freedom. Play requires the physical freedom to look messy, get dirty, see what's around the corner, and explore further down the block. It also requires trying and failing, acting silly, and saying or doing the wrong thing. If you value perfection, you don't have that kind of freedom, and you can't experience the pure joy and benefits of free play. I have good news for all the imperfect people out there, however: perfectionism is a terrible thing that stands in the way of progress and joy. The "perfect" is unattainable and thus depressing and self-defeating. Perfectionism deprives us of the ability to take chances, make mistakes, and play—all necessary steps for success. Perfectionists feel their accomplishments are never good enough, and this doesn't inspire them. Instead, it freezes them to never finish or—even worse—it exhausts and depletes them.

Perfectionism is rooted in fear—the fear that displays of imperfection will make us unworthy of acceptance and love. But the opposite is true. Our imperfections make us real and whole.

PRESCRIPTION

Create a Favorable Environment for Play
(Get Out of the Way!)

In the past, parents didn't have to work hard to create a favorable environment for their children to play in. Often, all they had to do was open the door. Now children have become accustomed to glittery customized dolls, cars that speak, hyperrealistic video games, and LEGO that comes with detailed instructions. But let me remind you: children love to play, it can cost nothing, you don't need a lot of stuff to make it happen, and you don't need any special instructions. Play doesn't even require toys. Commercial toys may actually get in the way of play. In general, the simpler the toys (which usually means those that are less expensive), the more divergent the play. Household items, old clothes, a stick, and whatever children find outside are ideal for play.

Interestingly, free play actually requires more focus from children, and more presence from parents who participate in their children's free play. And that's *real* presence—not checking your email on your phone. When an activity is unstructured, children (and participating parents) must be engaged intellectually and emotionally; otherwise, they would never be able to sustain that play. While children need no preparation for play, participating parents need to clear their decks.

Other crucial factors that contribute to creating a favorable environment for play are (1) limiting screen time (which we discussed in Chapter 5) and (2) not allowing homework to interfere with play.

PRESCRIPTION

Be Mindful of Homework

Homework has been steadily increasing over the last twenty years for younger students. But is there any good reason for the increase? According to research conducted in the United States since 1987, "no

strong evidence was found for an association between the homework–
achievement link and the outcome measure (grades as opposed to
standardized tests) or the subject matter (reading as opposed to
math)."[34] So we must ask ourselves, why take time away from something that is well proven to improve brain development in order to
force children to do something that has been shown to accomplish so
little?

If your intuition tells you that homework is being given mindlessly,
or to make a tiger teacher feel better, or to increase the school's
rankings, you're probably right. Ask yourself, *Is all this homework helping
or hindering my child's overall growth?* If you feel that it's not helping
and may even be hurting, see if there's any way to make the assignments more relevant, interesting, and/or fun. How can we connect
a homework project to CQ? Is there a way to use an assignment to
show your child how seemingly abstract concepts make a difference
in people's lives? For example, math concepts can be used to explain
everything from the family's shopping bills to unemployment statistics.

A lot of the homework I see is a relic of the nineteenth-century
school system and is in many ways irrelevant in the twenty-first century.
That kind of homework isn't just tedious, boring, and a turn off from
learning, it takes precious time away from real brain-boosting activities
such as play. Use your observations and intuition about homework.
How does your child look and behave as she's doing homework? Is it
too much for your child and he's getting turned off learning? Is it not
enough for your child and she's not being challenged? Children do best
when their learning is in the "zone of challenge"—not too easy, not too
hard, but just challenging enough to encourage problem solving and
learning. Homework can be a wonderful thing, but it's only one of many
ways children learn. The best learning is fun, based on real life, involves
trial and error, and is hands-on—that sounds like play to me!

PRESCRIPTION

Role Model the Value of Play

According to many physical anthropologists, humans are the most likely of all species to retain childlike qualities into adulthood—and this is a good thing![35] It means we get to continue to play. Play you should, especially in front of your child. If you don't have enough play in your life, reintroduce it. Take a music lesson, dance class, play a game you love on a regular basis, garden, hike, or simply explore for fun. The important thing here is to show your child that you, too, value exploration, play, creativity, trial and error, and fun!

PRESCRIPTION

Play in Nature

As a child, I found mindfulness through my curiosity and play in nature. Growing up, we didn't live in a beautiful natural setting, but we had a small backyard with dirt, a lot of bugs in the summer, a lot of snow in the winter, some scrawny trees, birds (crows), expansive prairie skies, and wind in the air year-round. The natural environment I had was all I needed. Almost all children have an intuitive curiosity for nature (before the tiger forces it out of them). Why do you think almost all babies stop crying when you take them outside? Most children love nature and everything in it—animals, trees, snow, sand, waves, and fresh air!

Since I had no tiger parents standing in my way, I was driven by my natural curiosity to spend hours and hours outside—seeing, hearing, smelling, tasting (yes—eating a lot of snow), and touching what was around me. Perhaps many of you reading this book had similar experiences growing up. What we didn't know at the time was that we were fine-tuning our external and internal senses and developing our intuition while we were "playing outside." Real play, as in "I lost track of time play," is a form of mindfulness. When we're absorbed in play, especially in nature, we go into a meditative state with all the associated benefits. Grass, dirt, bugs, snow, fresh air, trees, and birds were all I needed to meditate for hours. Of course, this behavior didn't last forever. What did last are my instincts to get outside—see the grass, smell the dirt, hear the leaves rustle and the birds chirp, have the wind touch my face, and taste the fresh air. I'm drawn to going outside, especially when I feel off balance or dysregulated (but I had forgotten this for many years). Being outside helps me notice and act on the signals Mother Nature is sending me before they become flashing lights, and I now know it and act on that knowledge. I try to get outside once a day—preferably for a walk alone with no distractions (that is, no cellphone). Sometimes even five or ten minutes can be enough. This practice (in addition to yoga, when I can get there) is my mindfulness.

Taking children out into nature is a great way to get them playing and enhancing mindfulness (and health, happiness, and self-motivation). I'm a firm believer that it's possible to suffer what Richard Louv dubbed "nature deficit disorder" in his 2005 book, *Last Child in the Woods*.[36] Although not recognized as an actual medical disorder—at least, not yet—my own experiences and those with my patients have convinced me that not enough time in nature can lead to all kinds of problems for children. In fact, ample research shows a link between time spent outside and our physical, cognitive, and emotional development.[37] Studies show that enjoying a natural setting such as a park, beach, wetland, or forest can reduce blood pressure, anxiety, and stress levels. Exposure to nature can help you sleep well and increase "vigor and liveliness." It can even boost your immune system.[38]

If exercise is good for you, exercise outdoors is even better. In 2008, researchers at Glasgow University put some science behind the idea.[39] The researchers looked at the effect on mental health of exercise in natural and non-natural environments. They observed people undertake physical activities such as walking, running, and cycling indoors and outdoors. They found that those who exercised outdoors had lower brain stress levels. The outdoor exercisers also experienced a nearly 50 percent improvement in mental health over the indoor exercisers. This improvement relates mainly to less severe mental health issues such as mild depression and insomnia.[40]

Being in nature makes people feel more alive.[41] According to a series of studies at the University of Rochester, being outdoors boosts vitality "above and beyond the influences of physical activity and social interactions."[42] According to the studies' lead author, Richard Ryan, "Research has shown that people with a greater sense of vitality don't just have more energy for things they want to do, they're also more resilient to physical illnesses. One of the pathways to health may be to spend more time in natural settings."[43]

I asked my patient Jasmine, a ballerina suffering from anxiety of "never knowing what to do" and feeling suffocated, how much time she spent outdoors each week. She looked at me incredulously at first; I imagined she was wondering how this question was relevant. But I asked her to just play along with me and count up the time she spent outdoors. She spent a few minutes calculating, then, looking a bit desperate, asked if "being in the car with the windows open" counted. "No," I answered. "OK then," Jasmine replied, "probably about sixty minutes Monday to Friday, and then maybe another hour on the weekend—so a total of about two hours of fresh air a week." Jasmine lives in a suburb and goes from her attached garage into a car for the ride to school. Basically, her time in nature consists of the Monday to Friday five-minute tree-lined walk from her mom's car to school (and back when her mom picks her up) and going in and out of her house. It's not enough. All of her exercise is indoors, and between ballet and academics, she is so busy that she often eats her meals and does her homework in the car. Jasmine's life is too busy, too structured, and too mindless. Jasmine felt suffocated because she had been bubble wrapped by her parents and had little chance to spend time in nature exploring, developing her intuition, following her curiosity, cultivating her intuition, and using all five of her external senses—everything needed to "know what to do" and adapt.

No Need to "Pencil It in" on Your Calendar— Just Play!

You don't have to schedule play into your child's life or set aside time to play with your child. Play is easy to incorporate into your everyday life. For example, toothbrushing in the morning can become a battle between the "bad guys," whose weapons are bacteria, and the "good guys," whose weapon is toothpaste. Getting dressed can become an Olympic sport with gold, silver, and bronze medals for the fastest times. When we're in a lineup or at a red light, my children and I often play a game we call "connecting," where we take three random things and come up with some kind of connection between them. Even homework supervision can be playful. Sometimes I put on my teacher's glasses and pretend that I'm evil "Mrs. Mean." When my children get a question wrong, Mrs. Mean cackles with delight, which my children find hysterical. When they get a question right, Mrs. Mean is devastated and has a tantrum, which they find equally hysterical.

In addition to these kinds of everyday play, you can also encourage play in order to understand your child's interests. As Plato said, "You can discover more about a person in an hour of play than in a year of conversation." I like to ask my children, "Is there something you want to try that you haven't yet? When I was your age, I used to ride my bike to the store, help make pancakes for breakfast, manage my own allowance, play and explore with wood, clay, etc. What would be fun for you to do?" I was surprised when my older son told me he wanted to "crack an egg" and my younger son said he wanted to make nachos and cheese!

Because many people have come to feel that free time is a waste of time, I also encourage parents to make sure their children have time to do "nothing." A young patient of mine was suffering from depression, and because he told me that being outside helped him relax, I suggested to his mother that he have some unstructured time outdoors. Her response? "What is my child going to do outside? Stand there looking at the clouds when he can be learning something?" Later that month, I had another patient referred to me for an assessment for ADHD. When I asked her what the concern was, she said, "My teacher noticed that I'm always distracted in class, looking out the window and staring at the clouds." Well, after the assessment I concluded that this young girl didn't have ADHD at all. She was just too busy and overprotected and really needed some time to just go outside and stare at the clouds!

CQ Developers in Play

In their groundbreaking book *The Innovator's DNA*, Jeff Dyer, Hal Gregersen, and Clayton Christensen identified five behaviors associated with the world's best innovators. Luckily, all of these behaviors, which I refer to as *CQ developers*, are the very things that children love to do, if given the opportunity. They're also a natural part of play, which means that we don't need any special training to do them!

CQ Developer #1: Encourage Observing

Children can spend a lot of time watching how things—often simple and mundane—happen. Whether they're moving sand from one pile to another, watching water run down a drain, or watching ants walk in a row, children are observing. When they carefully watch the world around them, children gain insights that can spark new ideas, new ways of doing things, and new ways of connecting things and ideas.

If children are shuffled from one structured activity to another, when will they have the time to observe the world? If they're constantly given instruction on how to do things, when will they have the ability to observe how things naturally happen, what interests them, what puzzles them, and how to satisfy their curiosity?

CQ Developer #2: Encourage Questioning

One of the best ways to develop critical-thinking skills is to ask *a lot* of questions. Consider Leonardo da Vinci—arguably one of history's greatest critical and creative thinkers—and his insatiable quest for learning:

> I roamed the countryside searching for the answers to things I did not understand. Why shells existed on the tops of mountains along with the imprints of coral and plant and seaweed usually found in the sea. Why the thunder lasts a longer time than that which causes it and why immediately on its creation the lightning becomes visible to the eye while thunder requires time to travel. How the various circles of water form around the spot which has been struck by a stone and why a bird sustains itself in the air. These questions and other strange phenomena engaged my thought throughout my life.[44]

Asking questions is something children do naturally and quite expertly—and questions occur when they feel free to play and explore. "Why is the sky blue? Why is the grass green? Why does the sun rise on this side and set on that side? Why do you have to go to work? Why do people have to die? Why, why, why …?"

Children who question anything and everything have a passion for challenging the status quo and pushing boundaries. Innovators have what is called a high *Q/A ratio*, "where questions (Q) not only outnumber answers (A) in a typical conversation, but are valued at least as highly as good answers."[45] I'd argue that the same applies to critical thinkers. In fact, I think it's fair to say that you can't be much of an innovator unless you're a critical thinker.

Overscheduling, memory drills, and endless practice are question killers. So too is the fear of being wrong. If you're afraid to make mistakes or you worry that asking a question will make you look foolish, you won't ask any.

Asking the right questions has been shown in research and anecdotally to have led to some of the biggest breakthroughs in science, business, technology, and global solutions. But what happens in a world where test scores and right answers are seen as key determinants of intelligence? I once heard a professor say that "being a professor these days is easy—students don't ask any questions!"

CQ Developer #3: Encourage Experimenting

All animals learn about the world through trial and error. I'm sure the first dolphin who used a sea sponge over his snout to forage for food on the ocean floor didn't get it right initially, but ultimately was pretty thrilled by his invention. Trial and error is important for children too: by trying a new experience, children learn (1) whether they're capable of doing it, (2) how to become capable of doing it, and (3) whether they like doing it enough to want to do it again. Remember the Dr. Seuss story *Green Eggs and Ham*, where Sam-I-Am harangues his friend to try green eggs and ham. He offered them in a box with a fox, in a house with a mouse, and in a boat with a goat, but the friend refused to try them. Sam-I-Am never gave up and eventually convinced his friend to experiment. Lo and behold, his friend discovered that he loved them.

By definition, experimenting requires trial and error, and that means making mistakes and even failing. Experimenting and making mistakes teaches children about the process of "figuring things out" and of success. Through mistakes and failure, children learn that not everything works out on the first or even the tenth try. Mistakes allow children an opportunity to stop and assess what they're doing and consider what they can change in order to succeed next time.

Failure that comes from experimenting isn't actually failure at all; it's a learning opportunity for eventual success. For example, when Edison tried to invent the light bulb, he failed 9,000 times. He said, "I didn't fail 9,000 times—I learned 9,000 ways not to make a light bulb."[46]

Children who understand that failure is a necessary aspect of learning actually perform better. Children who are shunned or punished for making mistakes may become afraid of making them. Those children may only attempt to do things they know they'll succeed at and thus won't "play." Children who are rewarded only when they're "right" won't learn to appreciate the value of mistakes, which will make them less likely to take risks and try new things.

CQ Developer #4: Encourage Associating

Associating involves connecting, reorganizing, and delivering known ideas in a new way. It's something tiger cubs have a hard time with because they often lack a variety of real-life experiences and the freedom to think beyond instructions. In a 1996 interview with *Wired* magazine, Steve Jobs talked about the importance of connecting and why there isn't more of it: "A lot of people in our industry haven't had very diverse experiences. So they don't have enough dots to connect, and they end up with very linear solutions without a broad perspective on the problem."[47]

In a 2005 commencement speech he gave at Stanford University, Jobs said, "You can't connect the dots looking forward; you can only connect them looking backwards. So you have to trust that the dots will somehow connect in your future."[48] Here's an example of how Steve Jobs connected his "dots." After dropping out of Reed College at the end of his first semester, Steve came back to audit a class in calligraphy. It wasn't a required class or a prerequisite (since he wasn't a Reed College student anymore). As Jobs put it, calligraphy had no "hope of any practical application in my life. It was beautiful, historical, artistically subtle in a way that science can't capture, and I found it fascinating."[49] It wasn't until years later that Jobs reconnected with his love for calligraphy and incorporated its graceful aesthetics into Apple product design.

CQ Developer #5: Encourage Networking

Networking involves connecting with a broad range of people. Although people in our networks may be like-minded, powerful connections occur when we network with those who have very different ideas from ours.

When people from diverse backgrounds and with different views connect, ideas are tested and new ideas emerge. If you've ever been stuck on a problem, you know that often running it by others is the ticket to a breakthrough.

Some children are natural networkers, going from classmate to classmate in the playground, while others tend to stick with the same few people. Either way, we know that allowing children to network results in an exchange of ideas and an appreciation for new ideas.

How much networking and collaboration do you think young students going to night tutoring schools do? For years, they're instructed in drills and facts, and spend every waking hour—even hours they shouldn't be awake—on perfecting those drills and memorizing those facts.

In the Western world, children usually don't spend a lot of time doing one thing. But they may be putting in numerous hours engaged in a variety of activities, such as piano, rowing, ballet, and math. In many cases, these activities are highly structured and directed by an instructor or coach, and that limits or eliminates the real-life networking and collaboration that could occur.

Anyone in the business field will tell you that strong social skills are key to strong networks and collaboration. Have you seen the brilliant HSBC ad declaring that "in the future, business will be social"? I think the future has come. The next chapter is exactly about our fundamental need and desire to be social.

Chapter 7

HUMANS ARE SOCIAL BEINGS

I had the heartbreaking, yet inspiring, experience of being with my father-in-law during the last moments of his life. He had suffered for years with painful prostate cancer and died just four months after my husband and I were married. When I looked into his eyes as he took his last breaths, I could feel the legacy he was leaving behind. A millworker, he never changed the world in any big way. But he was a man of integrity, with strong ethics, principles, and values. As a result, in his small community he was a leader who set a strong moral tone with far-reaching effects. Hundreds and hundreds of people—far more than we expected—came to his funeral. It seemed as though they had all come to say the same thing: thank you. In his short life of just sixty years, my father-in-law managed to touch all of these lives. Some noted what he did for them: "he helped me get a job," "he stood up for me at the mill," and "he lent me money when I needed it." However, others, many of whom my husband had never even met, noted what he stood for: "he always did what was right," "he cared about people," and "he was a man of character." At his funeral, I saw firsthand and up close the most important thing a human life can be remembered for: an individual's contribution to his world and community.

Although my children have never met their grandfather, whenever we meet someone who knew him, they immediately hear about the qualities he's remembered for. I know my children feel the imprint of their grandfather through these comments and stories, and I believe these stories add to my children's own positive feelings about community and contribution.

When we pass on, almost all of us, even if we don't recognize it now, will want to be remembered for the bonds we shared with others and for having done some good in our lives. What I'm talking about here is the very deepest of human desires: an intense need to connect with others and have a purpose in life. In fact, these are cited as the main reasons people have children. We all want to leave the message that "I was here," and that message is for our loved ones, our community, and the world around us. I suspect that most people, in the last moments of their life, consider whether they're leaving this world better than when they found it.

Dolphins, like humans, are highly social and have a strong sense of community. The centerpiece of the dolphin way of life is the pod—a rich social community of dolphins who live, work, and play together. When a member of their community is sick or injured, dolphins will stay with that member, often swimming below them and pushing them to the surface to breathe.

Sometimes, several dolphin pods join together to form a super pod with as many as 1,000 dolphins traveling together. They bond socially, hunt, and play together, and they protect and help other dolphin species (more than forty dolphin species exist, ranging from the four-foot-long Hector dolphin of New Zealand to the twenty-foot-long orca of the Arctic and Antarctic). This is true even if these other dolphin species look different and don't communicate in the same way. Dolphins also show a sense of community in their eating habits: they take no more than they need and share their meals with dolphins in their pod and other pods and even with non-mammals such as tuna.

Helping one another and forming sophisticated aquatic alliances within their species and other species is all part of the dolphin way of life. Consider the following example. In 2008 in New Zealand, a group of whales had somehow beached themselves.[1] Many locals came to help and were successful in pushing the giants back into the water. But because the whales were unfamiliar with their surroundings, they ended up directly back on the beach—stranded and in serious peril. People kept trying to help, but the whales kept heading back to the beach. Eventually, both the whales and their human helpers became exhausted and were close to giving up. That's when Moko the dolphin, known throughout the town for showing up to play with swimmers, showed up. Moko swam directly to the distressed whales, a signal that he was ready to help. This time, after the whales were again pushed off the sand into the water, they moved into position behind Moko and he led them (proudly, it seemed) back to sea, while cheers erupted from the astonished humans on the beach.

Dolphins have also been known to help people. A fourteen-year-old boy who couldn't swim fell off his father's boat and was drowning when a dolphin suddenly appeared. The dolphin lifted the boy to the surface and pushed him close enough to his father's boat so that the father could grab the boy and pull him onboard. In another case, dolphins created a protective ring around a man being preyed on by a shark, staying with the man until the shark left and human help arrived.[2]

During the first years of a young dolphin's life, parents prioritize a sense of community and hunting. Why is community connection prioritized as much as hunting skills? It's a big ocean out there, and dolphins have learned that their best chance to survive and prosper is to work together with their pod and even to work with other pods when needed. In fact, evidence suggests that dolphins have more success raising their young—losing fewer to predators or other calamities—when they have strong relationships with other pod members.[3] Even before birth, pod members referred to as "aunties" help pregnant dolphins stay healthy by sharing food with them and assisting them in the birthing process.

What Is Community?

We're born into the world of our parents, but for most of our lives, we must survive and thrive in a world of our own. Both worlds, of childhood and adulthood, are dominated by social interactions.

A *community* is "a social, religious, occupational, or other group sharing common characteristics or interests and perceived or perceiving itself as distinct in some respect from the larger society within which it exists."[4] A community can also simply be "your people" or "your pod"—those you care for and share your life with.

Children learn how others cope with struggles and disappointments from their community. They also learn the value of humility, resilience, and problem solving. They learn how members of the community can help others who are stuck or have made mistakes. They learn about having fun as a group. They experience the joy of sharing one's successes with others and the comfort of receiving support during setbacks.

A community provides an environment within which rich social bonds can form—including those of friends, mentors, and role models. The only way to learn essential social skills is by trying them out. In a community, through trial and error, young people will quickly learn the downsides of being too competitive, perfectionistic, overconfident, entitled, and self-righteous. They'll learn to communicate, collaborate, and resolve conflict. They'll learn to be accountable for their actions and how to trust, respect, and be fair to others. Thinking beyond oneself is the essence of a community, the very definition of a contribution.

Although it may seem paradoxical, the very skills needed for independence and individual achievement develop within the structure and security of the community. Growing up in a community teaches children how to eventually find, create, and nurture their own communities, regardless of their stage in life, their occupation, or their address. We build our identity in our community; it's the place where we start finding answers to fundamental questions such as Who am I? What is my place in this world? What am I about? What do I want to do with my life? The answers to these questions aren't found through solitary functioning; they're found through the experience of collective identity and in relation to the real world. When children become teenagers or young adults, they may "try on" various identities and move in and out of their communities. They might see what it feels like to be a rebel, a skater, a snob, an athlete, an academic, or a nerd until, eventually, they find their own identity. They may claim that they don't care what anyone thinks, but it would be a mistake to believe them. The whole point of defining our role in society and our relationship with others is to build a *social* identity.

Families need to be communities, but they aren't always. Cara, a fifteen-year-old patient of mine, was sexually abused by her uncle. After much angst, she decided to disclose the trauma to her family, only to face an initial "sealing over" of the abuse by them. Distraught, she turned to drugs and ran away from home.

My heart broke for her, and I worked with the police to find her. After two weeks of no word, I feared the worst. Yet, all the time Cara was missing, she had found a sense of belonging with a truly extraordinary community. She ended up on the Downtown Eastside of Vancouver, an area notorious for crime, drug use, and prostitution. However, it has incredibly strong communities too. There, Cara met a young woman who had a similar story and introduced her to several other women who could relate to Cara in some way (many of them were prostitutes dealing with their own addictions). These women took care of Cara; they kept her safe and gave her shelter and food. They listened to her and didn't judge her, and they guided Cara away from their own mistakes and towards her own home. Once back in treatment, Cara told me that she felt good when she was with these women. Because of her bonds with them, Cara decided to turn her life around and focus on the future instead of the past. Cara went back to school and is a now a passionate and outspoken women's rights advocate working in the Downtown Eastside. She now tells me that despite the trauma of her past, she is happy.

What Is Contribution?

We sometimes think of contribution as something reserved for socialite housewives or selfless churchgoers. Nothing could be further from the truth. All of us are hardwired to give. When we contribute, we're rewarded with a feeling of well-being and joy. Biology needs us to contribute for our very survival; when contribution isn't part of our lives, we become off balance, unwell, and unhealthy. Like playing, if you're not giving, you're dying.

Generation Y studies tell us that today's youth value money and status more than any other generation did before them.[5] At the same time, today's youth are also considered among the least motivated; their sense of entitlement is high, and their ability to "put in the hard work" is at an all-time low. If money and status are clearly not enough to motivate today's youth, what is?

Contribution. I believe working towards a greater purpose is seriously undervalued as a human motivator, especially by parents. Just like social bonding and community, we know that contribution is important, but we parents sometimes forget to honor it. Consider the messages on Hallmark cards and the remarks at wedding toasts. Compliments that really touch the heart are those that say we're "caring," have "been there" for others, or were "always willing to help." "You make the world a better place" is one of the highest compliments a person can receive.

Marketers know that people value contribution, so it's no surprise that this idea has become part of numerous marketing campaigns. Whether the business is a car mechanic, a local market, a law firm, or a corporation, common slogans are "because we care," "we make a difference," and "we believe." The University of San Francisco has a wonderful slogan: "Change the world from here."

Laura is the daughter of a friend of mine, and she's also a talented musical performer. Yet, despite her immense talent, Laura was struggling with her motivation and practice. She wasn't practicing her music and vocals enough and generally had a "bad attitude." Laura seemed motivated by some form of contribution because she loved to entertain and make others happy. But her parents were perplexed as to why her motivation to perform was waning, especially since she was getting rave reviews. Her father told me about Laura's most powerful and poignant performance—a performance Laura needed absolutely no coaxing or prodding to prepare for and one that she delivered superbly. The play she performed was on a topic that Laura truly connected with—the story of a young girl who fought for her right to an education despite all odds. In fact, Laura was so moved by the play that she decided to visit the playwright, who was an old woman living in a nursing home. It turns out that the playwright had helped Laura deal with a struggle she was facing in her own life. Laura had had access to a good education, but there was something in her life that she felt she had to fight for that the play helped her work out. Laura simply wanted to say "thank you" to the playwright for the contribution she had made to Laura's life. From this experience, Laura realized why her motivation had stalled: she wanted to do more than "entertain" people; she wanted to "move" people like the playwright had moved her. She wanted to change lives through her art. She wanted to "make a difference."

Contributing to the world through our unique gifts is the ultimate motivator. I prescribe contribution to all my patients because I know it will release some much-needed dopamine in their brains. Just writing a check and sending in a donation is satisfying. But it's even more satisfying to use our unique talents to contribute to the world. Think of superheroes. Every superhero wants to save the world—that's the essence of the superhero, isn't it? Each superhero has a special power that gives him or her the ability to uniquely contribute. Like all of us, superheroes have weaknesses that stand in the way of their contribution—a truly invulnerable superhero would be boring. The fact that many have an alter ego who lives an ordinary life tells us that anybody can be great and have superhero qualities. Superheroes represent our best values (such as justness, virtue, and caring), which is why the stories tend to be timeless and have universal appeal. Who doesn't want to rise above their everyday concerns and do something truly beneficial for others?

People often contribute to their own communities through their work. Doctors do it by helping people become healthy, teachers do it by shaping the minds of the next generation, and journalists do it by digging for the truth. I've noticed that those who like their job because it allows them to give back often received meaningful help from others in the past that contributed to their own growth and success.

Parents often say, "It doesn't matter what you do, as long as you do your best." Why? Because doing your best *does* matter. If you try to be the best you can be at something, that simple fact can inspire others to be their best—and that's contribution. So too is making a difference, fulfilling your purpose, and leaving the world better than you found it.

The Biological Rewards of Community and Contribution

Interacting and connecting socially makes us experience well-being and joy. The sense of well-being and joy is biology rewarding us for something that's important for our survival. Social interaction and social bonding both boost dopamine in our brains, but social bonding is rewarded more. Why is one social activity rewarded more than the other? From a biological perspective, social interaction is a step in the right direction to our survival (meeting and interacting with others is important), but social bonding builds a healthy community—and healthy communities are essential to our survival. It's like the difference between dating and falling in love. Meeting and/or flirting on a date releases some dopamine, but falling in love (which might lead to offspring that would expand the community) releases a massive amount of dopamine. When oxytocin (a "feel-good" hormone released when we cuddle, hug, and kiss) is added to the mix, feelings of deep contentment and comfort are the result.

If you're not yet convinced that humans are completely social animals, just spend some time with teenagers and you'll see how strongly social behaviors are hardwired into their developing brains. From puberty onward, they become completely consumed with social behaviors, such as who's doing what and with whom. For the young brain, social interaction is a powerful amplifier of reward, and peer group interactions increase dopamine release. Consider how thrilled teenagers feel when they're invited to a party and how gloomy they feel when they're left out. Some brain scan studies suggest that youth brains react to peer exclusion similar to how they would react to threats of physical harm or to starvation.[6] In other words, adolescents may perceive social rejection as a threat to their very existence. This last point may make it easier to understand why teenagers react to social ups and downs, whether in person, online, or in their imagination, as if their very lives depended upon them.

Social bonding is so all-important for happiness that it's been shown to be even more powerful than the basic necessities of life. A study carried out from 2005 to 2010—and covering 155 countries—by researchers at the University of Illinois found that people felt well-being and realized self-actualization even if their basic needs were not fulfilled, as long as they continued to have strong, positive relationships with other people.[7] Even in times of war, when the basic necessities of life can become limited and security needs are unfulfilled, people have reported a sense of happiness as long as they maintained positive social connections. In fact, the study found that extreme situations in which people lack the necessities of life and face ongoing danger can strengthen social bonds; for this reason, some who have lived through a terrible trauma such as war have described that time as one of the best in their lives.

The same study found that people were happier if the needs of others in their society were also fulfilled.[8] In other words, an individual's satisfaction depends not only on his or her quality of life but also on that of others. Yes, of course, we're built to gather, protect, compete, and establish our own individual security, but we're also built to connect socially and care about our community. There's now actual science to support the old adage, "the more you give, the more you get." A 2008 study by Harvard Business School professor Michael Norton and colleagues found that giving money to someone else increased participants' happiness more than spending it on themselves.[9] A 2006 study found that just thinking about giving to others stimulates the same parts of the brain activated by the pleasures of eating and sex.[10] MRIs tracking the brain showed that donating money to charity activates the brain's reward center, which we know causes dopamine-mediated well-being and joy.[11]

Contribution can actually prolong our lives. A study on the elderly showed that those who gave emotional support to their spouse or practical help to others in their community (friends, relatives, neighbors) had a lower risk of dying over five years than those who did not.[12] A University of California, Berkeley study of seniors found that those who volunteered at two or more organizations were 44 percent less likely to die over a five-year period (factors such as age, smoking, other negative health habits, general health, and exercise patterns were all controlled for).[13] It won't kill you to lend a hand—but it may kill you not to.

Developing CQ Through Community and Contribution

James Watson and Francis Crick were just two of the many people trying to uncover the structure of human DNA in the 1950s. In 1953 they made scientific history by becoming the first to identify the famous double helix structure of DNA, which was groundbreaking for molecular biology and genetics. What makes the Watson/Crick discovery so interesting is that Crick was a physicist and Watson was a zoologist—two occupations that seem far removed from chemistry and human biology. But the two pushed, challenged, debated, disagreed, tried to convince each other, and eventually agreed on something remarkable.

Working alone, it's much harder to come up with new solutions or even to test the ones you already have. But in a team, the debate among people with diverse backgrounds is what produces the best ideas. In his memoirs, Crick wrote that he doubts he would ever have identified the double helix structure working on his own.[14]

Two components of CQ are collaboration and communication. To collaborate and communicate, you need social skills—the ability to get along with others, to express yourself effectively and influence others, and to work with people you may not necessarily like. Social skills can make the difference between success and failure—both in school and long after graduation. A child who's well liked at school is generally a child who will do well in the long run. But a socially awkward child is going to have a much harder time making friends, keeping friends, and working on projects with other students. In fact, research shows that kindergarten students' ability to make new friends and be accepted by their classmates predicts how much they'll participate in the classroom, and even how independently they'll work on academic tasks.[15] In other words, the more social skills a child has, the more that child is able to learn independently.

Experiencing social challenges allows children to be spontaneous, to negotiate, to be assertive, to diversify, and to adapt. Social interactions open up opportunities for discussing and resolving upsetting, emotional situations. All of these skills promote creativity and critical thinking, the other two Cs in CQ. When children are always practicing some narrow skill set, or dropped off and picked up from an activity where a teacher instructs them the entire time, they can't learn the life skills that only happen in real-life social situations. I once overheard a mother bemoaning the fact that many of the children in her neighborhood were younger than her ten-year-old son. She said, "He has no choice but to play with children younger than himself, and that worries me because he's not learning anything. I prefer when he plays with children the same age or older than him, then he can at least pick up new skills." She was dead wrong. Yes, a child who plays with older children may learn some new skills, such as how to throw a ball better or some new vocabulary. However, children who play with younger children learn *many* important social skills. In fact, they learn compassion and empathy, which are essential to emotional intelligence and success in life. The older child must learn to read younger children's non-verbal cues and help them overcome obstacles. Equally important, the older child must effectively explain new concepts to children with less verbal understanding. There's nothing like having to explain something to a younger child to solidify your own knowledge or expose areas that need development.

Interacting with people of all ages in your community also teaches CQ. We learn values such as accountability and responsibility; the importance of keeping our word and meeting our commitments; and how to earn the respect, regard, and admiration of others (and how quickly one can lose the respect, regard, and admiration of others through unethical or unprincipled behaviors). Children with high CQ value citizenship and understand the importance of belonging and contributing to the community.

We're at a pivotal point in human history, when our activities are changing the planet and its ecosystems more rapidly than in the past. With seven billion people and counting, our massive footprint will only increase, and so too will the severity of the problems and changes we face. If ever there was a time to come together as a community to solve our problems, it's now. The challenges of the next generation are daunting, and the decisions they make will be critical. Thankfully, as we've seen, we're hardwired to care, share, and cooperate. So, now, more than ever, we need to follow what we are naturally built to do.

Tigers Ignore Community and Contribution

Even though social bonding is in our nature, we often forget this truth. I see it all the time—people who forget or minimize our need for social connection then wonder why they feel depressed, anxious, and tired.

Tigers don't see their environments as communities but rather as arenas, some big and some small, but all defined by individual performance. In an arena, everyone competes and only those that can help you "win"—that is, gain an immediate goal like acing the next test or competition—hold value. This thinking often leads tiger cubs to be overly competitive and lacking in important social skills, such as collaboration and communication.

Tiger cubs are so accustomed to being in the arena that they tend to see others as competition—their classmates, teammates, even their own siblings. Instead of sharing in the joy of a sibling's, a friend's, or a cousin's accomplishments, tiger cubs may feel nervous or jealous because their lives are punctuated with a constant fear of not being the best. Because they grow up in an environment where they're rewarded for what they do and not who they are, they internalize the belief that their accomplishments define who they are and fail to develop a true sense of identity.

Whether they mean to or not, tiger parents often segregate their children from others. Tiger cubs are often busy with school-work and in age-defined activities run by hired adults. They don't have a lot of time for friends or family (including grandma and grandpa, even if they live nearby). The role of friends, cousins, aunts, uncles, and grandparents is diminished because tiger cubs are involved mainly in activities that will help them be "the best." Sadly, as a result, tiger cubs lose out on opportunities for positive role modeling, guiding, mentoring, and other cross-generational interactions. Tiger cubs lack access to a variety of perspectives. They often learn in isolation or from a few individuals, many of whom may be paid to teach them—such as tutors—and who likely have similar worldviews as their parents.

A life without real social connections is very lonely. Now, loneliness may not sound like the worst thing in the world—especially if you're sitting in a penthouse with a six-figure salary. After all, it's lonely at the top, right? If this is your view, let me tell you: loneliness can kill you. Let's start with the most extreme form of loneliness, solitary confinement.

Solitary confinement represents one of the great ironies in the history of human cruelty. The first prison with solitary cells was built in the 1820s, and the intention of solitary confinement was to provide a more humane way of housing criminals. Prior to this time, criminals were housed in overcrowded jails ruled by gangs and marked by humiliation and danger. As brutal as over-crowding conditions were, jailers soon found out that being alone was even worse: prisoners in solitary confinement were going "mad." Today, the harmful consequences of solitary confinement are extremely well documented. These include sleep disturbances, anxiety, depression, panic, rage, loss of control, paranoia, hallucinations, self-mutilation, cognitive dysfunction, and complete psychological breakdown.[16] What was once conceived as a humanitarian gesture is now one of the most fearsome threats in the hands of jailors and torturers around the world.

It turns out that emotional isolation is ranked just as high a risk factor for mortality as smoking.[17] In the 1950s, therapist Frieda Fromm-Reichmann laid the groundwork for how loneliness affects a person—a topic so complex that we still haven't thoroughly understood it. Loneliness isn't just a feeling. It corrodes the whole body, like a disease. It alters hormonal signals and pathways that can cause damage to the systems they control, such as gene regulation. Prolonged isolation can worsen many conditions, such as Alzheimer's disease, obesity, cancer, and heart disease. For example, research shows that tumors will metastasize faster in lonely people.[18]

Loneliness is more than physical isolation. Fromm-Reichmann defined *loneliness* as the prolonged desire for intimacy.[19] Even a person who is surrounded by people all day long can still experience true loneliness. UCLA research on loneliness has found that as many as 30 percent of Americans don't feel significantly close to any person in their life.[20] A 2010 AARP study of adults forty-five years and older found that one in three felt lonely for prolonged periods, an increase from one in five in the early 2000s.[21]

A 2006 UCLA study showed that the neural systems activated by physical pain and social rejection overlap.[22] The study involved a game of "cyberball," in which three players—one human and two computer programs—tossed a ball to one another. (The human player thought that the other two players were people.) After the ball was tossed back and forth among the players for a while, the two computer programs started to "ignore" the person, and threw the ball back and forth to each other alone. When this happened, MRI scans of the person showed that this rejection activated the same part of the brain associated with physical pain.

The "Quarter Life Crisis of the Tiger"

Ava, a lawyer and an accomplished pianist, was twenty-nine and the mother of a three-month-old when she came to see me. "My baby isn't attractive and cries more than other babies," she told me. If you didn't know Ava, you might think *Oh come on, get real*. But unfortunately for Ava, the feeling that her baby wasn't perfect was *very* real.

After working with new moms for ten years, I can tell you that the more competitive—and thus more perfectionistic and lonely—the tiger, the greater the post-partum adjustment. Nothing requires more humility, tolerance of imperfection, thinking on your feet, and help from your community than the first few weeks of being a new parent. Ava was having a very hard time. "I have always been the best at whatever I do," she told me. "I really don't know how to do anything imperfectly." Then she went on to confess that not a single person had come over to make her food, watch the baby, or invite her over like the other moms she knew.

It soon became clear that so many of Ava's problems stemmed from the fact that she was used to winning. She couldn't adjust to the real world, for which a lifetime of tutors and daily rehearsal had left her completely unprepared. Of course, Ava spent a lot of time in childhood dealing with exam and performance stress, but she had spent no time dealing with general life stress—those tedious and often ambiguous things that frustrate us, such as doing household chores, juggling responsibilities, and working in a team.

Ava also grew up believing that getting good grades and winning competitions made her special and somehow exempted her from having to do regular, ordinary tasks. Surely, she shouldn't waste her precious time doing dishes at home when she had to study or practice. Now, as an adult, these real-life responsibilities were adding up fast and getting in her way.

Tragically, Ava was having difficulty embracing her own child without comparing her child to others. Even her few friends found this rejection a real turn off. But then, Ava really didn't know how not to compete and establish close bonds with others, especially among her own peers—including her own husband. It's not hard to imagine that people who interacted with her just didn't like her.

Her perfectionism and need to be on top also made her harshly self-critical. She was particularly critical of her appearance and body after the baby was born. She spent a lot of time and money she didn't have to get back into "shape" and still felt miserable. Yet the most distressing thing for Ava was that she expected all her childhood hard work and sacrifice to "pay off," as if someone were keeping score in a competition called life. I see this type of phenomenon often and have come to call it the "quarter life crisis of the tiger."

After months of therapy and a lot of positive change on Ava's part, she burst into tears in my office one day. She told me that she had come to realize that her childhood was lost on the wrong things. Her pursuit of individual achievement at the expense of all else had cost her dearly. But, thankfully, her despair was short-lived. In her newfound dolphin spirit, Ava was determined that her daughter's childhood would be different. She would focus more on helping her daughter develop social bonds and strive for her best self rather than encourage her daughter to compete against others. She wanted her daughter to thrive during life's journey through ever-changing waters, not to win within the confines of an arena, and she realized that her child needed a community for that.

With so many young people today growing up to be like the Ava who first walked in my door, as "Gen Entitled," we must ask ourselves this: Is a social life or social status a substitute for social bonds? Are we losing our sense of citizenship, sharing, and caring that's so vital for positive character development and leadership? Who will help make the world a better place? Isn't it the role of parents to help their children develop a positive character? Yes it is, *and* yes you can!

PRESCRIPTION

Create a Favorable Environment for Community and Contribution

Create a community for your children to grow up in—a community built upon values such as trust, respect, responsibility, empathy, integrity, and humility. Your community should be made up of people you would turn to when you need help. Depending on your circumstances, your community could be all of your family or none of your family. It could include a mentor, old friends, colleagues, or parents of your children's friends. Each community member may play a different role in your life. I can't tell you how many times I've seen a grandparent, aunt, friend, or teacher/coach be a pivotal person in a youth's life when the parent–child relationship has become strained. Indeed, sometimes the greatest lessons in life come from a loving and well-respected non-parent adult (or sibling).

A community is based on quality relationships, not a quantity of people. Quality relationships are the people who would visit you in the hospital if you were sick. Although you may have hundreds of Facebook "friends," how many would be there for you when you need them? A community member is someone you feel nurtures you and who you nurture back. Living in a community is not about living a life "for other people"—that's a one-way relationship. It's about giving to and receiving from others.

Many children parented by tigers don't have the time to connect with others, including their grandparents, aunts, uncles, cousins, or the friends who are supposed to be part of their community. I've heard many grandmothers say, "I never get to see my grandson because he's always so busy." If you've made a conscious decision to keep your children away from a certain person because you don't like that person's influence on your children, that's your choice as a parent. However, if children are being deprived of developing and participating in their community simply because they're too busy, then you must reconsider how busy they are. Children who are shuffled from school to sports to music lessons may see, interact, and compete with others, but they're left with little time to develop meaningful social bonds. So, freeing up your and your children's time to spend with your community is a must. And there's an added benefit for you: the great thing about living in a community is that you often have far less work to do as a parent.

PRESCRIPTION

Be a Role Model for Community and Contribution

The best role model for community and contribution is you. When you show that you value community and contribution, you display true leadership and people notice and remember, especially your children. If you want your children to value meaningful social bonds, a connection to their communities, and a greater purpose in life, you must try your best to value all of those things yourself.

If we value quality relationships, our children will internalize that knowledge and be better able to establish such relationships in their own lives. If we want our children to have meaningful friendships, we need to have meaningful friendships. If we want our children to get rid of meaningless relationships, we need to get rid of our own meaning-less relationships. If we want our children to surround themselves with authentic, nurturing people, then we need to surround ourselves with authentic, nurturing people. Just like what we do influences who we are, who we spend time with also influences who we are.

Given this, it's easy to understand that being around positive people inspires us to be positive. This type of effect doesn't just come from the words a person says, but also how the words are said and the energy in the room at the time. The human heart's electromagnetic field can be measured several feet away from our bodies and can be sensed by others. Thus, this energetic system plays an important role in communicating physical, emotional, and interpersonal information between individuals.[23] Some individuals can have a calming and moti-vating presence by bringing their stable and organized electromagnetic field closer to someone whose field is less coherent. And stable fields lead to stable heart rhythms, which help the brain be creative and solve problems! It may sound a bit like the Jedi "force," but it's science!

PRESCRIPTION

Teach Values and Positive Character

At a recent dinner party I attended, guests were discussing the usual topics that keep parents up at night—schools, activities, curfews, and how our children will support themselves when they're even-tually out on their own. Someone told a story about a young man who made a small fortune selling relatively outdated technology to seniors. To my surprise, some of the parents around the dinner table applauded this young man's business sense; one pronounced it "brilliant." I disagreed. "To me, it's unethical," I said. Another parent spoke up. "There are two types of people in this world," he proclaimed, "those who screw others, and those who get screwed. Which one do you want your child to be?"

The question surprised me; I had never seen the world divided up quite that way. But this man insisted on an answer, so I gave it a try. I had a fleeting vision of my children looking very much like many of my financially "successful" patients: miserable, chasing some unknown prize, with no true friends, trying to numb their own thoughts and feelings, and unable to even look themselves in the eye. So, I said, "No. Screwing or being screwed is *not* the only choice. Being unprincipled serves no one. In fact, screwing others is completely incompatible with *true* success."

Of course, that comment was based solely on my personal experience, so as soon as I got home, I made it my mission to *prove* that it's possible to be simultaneously happy (not getting screwed) and ethical (not screwing others), and still be successful. To me, that's capital-S success in the twenty-first century—the ability to be healthy, happy, and successful via the moral character of a true leader. These are the qualities that can make the world a better place—or at least definitely not make it a worse place.

I found a wealth of information, research, and case studies that supported my conclusion. In fact, a lot of evidence shows that a strong moral character is not only an important part of life, but also an absolute prerequisite for true leadership and twenty-first-century success.[24] You can't have lasting success in this highly connected, social world without a strong moral compass, which includes integrity, responsibility, and a true sense of value for others. I wasn't interested in raising my children to screw others or get screwed.

Although many parents feel this way, they don't necessarily act accordingly because they are just too busy or too distracted. For some reason, moral character (and happiness) is considered a given. Parents say, "Well, of course, my child has to be ethical in every way" or "Absolutely, if my child had no values, that would be my biggest failure as a parent." In many cases, it's like saying, "Of course, good health is important" while eating unhealthy food and living an imbalanced life. Do you ever wonder why we adults (parents, teachers, coaches, and tutors) spend a lot of time teaching our children how to play an instrument, compete in a sport, and do homework, but little time teaching them the importance of social values and ethics? If being at the top of the class defines your child's self-esteem, she won't have any self-esteem when she's no longer the top student. If being a top athlete defines your child's self-esteem, that won't last either. A child's values last forever. Some parents might say that the process of learning how to play an instrument, compete in a sport, or do homework already teaches children social values and ethics. These activities will teach children the importance of discipline and hard work, but they won't teach the following crucial values: showing respect for those who are different or have nothing to offer you; doing the right thing when no one is looking and it doesn't count for anything; and being responsible to your community and the world you live in.

Values are actually among the most powerful of parenting tools. Values are what create meaning in our lives and shape our vision of the future, which brings us a greater sense of well-being. Strong values are linked to all kinds of success-related outcomes, and just thinking of values relieves stress! When we think about values, we're contemplating life's purpose and the resonance and dissonance of our behaviors with what really matters. This contemplation moves us from lower brain "mindless" reaction to our environment to higher brain "mindful" interaction with our environment. Consider the results of a 2005 UCLA study on stress, in which groups of individuals were subjected to stressful tasks in a lab. Prior to the stress tests, one group was asked to reflect on personal values that were meaningful to them, while the other groups were not. The group that reflected on meaningful personal values had lower levels of stress indicators such as cortisol (a stress hormone) in their bodies.[25]

I've seen the positive effects of value affirmation in my own clinic. Jaden was struggling with the issue of bullying at his school. He was not the target of bullying, but his neighbor down the street, Ravi, was. Jaden and Ravi were not great friends as they had different interests— Jaden was a real social sports kid and Ravi was into his gadgets and books, but Jaden liked Ravi. When Ravi was teased, it bothered Jaden so much that he began skipping gym class because he just couldn't see it anymore. Jaden thought of stepping in to defend Ravi, but felt scared he would become the next target. In one of our sessions, I could see Jaden was becoming really stressed and stuck, so we put aside the issues related to bullying. I simply took a clean sheet of paper and asked him to tell me about his values, and he responded with "friends and peace." Since he was only twelve, I wrote a list of common values, such as responsibility, fairness, empathy, and courage, and asked him to rank from one to ten how important each one was to him. He gave them all high marks of eight, nine, or ten. I then asked him to rank how he was *living according to these values,* and he ranked "responsibility" a four and "courage" a two. Jaden knew why he ranked these so low and so did I—he immediately felt unstuck and decided to talk to his school principal about the bullying.

Scrapbooking as a Way to Discover What Matters in Life

I'm one of those parents who never could get organized enough to make a scrapbook. I always envied the beautiful, colorful, and art-filled scrapbooks many mothers I knew would make for their children. I asked one friend why she goes through so much effort to make scrapbooks. Scrapbooking takes a lot of time, so what was her *real* motivation? She said, "I want to capture the special moments." "But *why* do you want to capture the special moments?" She responded, "I want my children to know what's important in life." Aha! I got it, and so did she. We looked at each other in one of those "that's a great idea" moments. She went on to change her scrapbook titles from "Disneyland" and "Birthday Party" to "Trust," "Fairness," "Responsibility," "Citizenship," "Respect," and "Caring."

I have no scrapbook supplies in my house, so I chose to create a "figurative scrapbook" (a continual discussion about what's important in life) with my children. Every so often, we add a "page"—usually just a brief conversation about a value that's important in our family. For example, my son came home and said, "Mom, I scored three goals in soccer today." I responded, "Good work! What did your teammates do that showed you that they trusted you? How did you treat them back in a fair way?" After the brief chat, I asked my son to describe a visual (or draw a picture) of what trust and fairness look like, and we then put that visual into our "scrapbook."

Our scrapbook also includes a "better world" category. For example, when my five-year-old asked me why he had to start kindergarten, I asked him what he thought the reason was. He offered a string of responses: "… to learn and become smart … to make friends … to a get a job one day …" To all of these I said, "Yes, and then what?" Eventually, he said "… to make the world a better place." "Yes, my dear child," I said, "you are going to kindergarten so that you can become smart, be happy, and grow into a leader that may someday make the world a better place … but first let's go to the bathroom so there are no accidents today!"

Creating a Gratitude Journal

A gratitude journal is a wonderful way to guide your child towards valuing community and contribution, in addition to improving health and happiness. I ask a number of my patients to use this journal—even the tough-looking teenage rebels on probation—and it's profoundly effective.

A gratitude journal is a diary where one writes down things that one is grateful for; it usually includes thoughts on community and contribution. The journal can be a highly effective ingredient in the development of

continued

neuroplasticity towards happiness. It asks the writer to pay close attention to the things that are positive in his or her life, and that may be why it works so well. Countless studies exist on the beneficial effects of gratefulness, such as an improved sense of happiness, personal growth, better social relationships, better sleep, less depression, less stress, and better coping skills.[26] *Time* magazine did a comprehensive review of the subject of gratefulness and concluded that "people who describe themselves as feeling grateful ... tend to have higher vitality and more optimism, suffer less stress, and experience fewer episodes of clinical depression than the population as a whole."[27]

Not surprisingly, research has shown that people who used gratitude journals felt better about their lives and reported fewer symptoms of illness.[28]

Chapter 8

A DOLPHIN PARENTING TOOLKIT

As soon as a baby orca is born, instead of being lifted to the surface to take its critical first breath of air, its mother gently nudges the newborn towards the surface while modeling swimming motions, thus encouraging independence right away. Despite this immediate message of self-reliance, the orca mother remains closely connected to her young, who rarely leave her side.

Orcas also take their young close to beaches and even beach them on shore, allowing them to "figure out for themselves" how to get back to open water, all the while staying nearby to guide and support these efforts. Orca mothers have been observed teaching their young how to catch fish off the Alaskan coast: the mothers chase the fish and keep the fish close while their young work at grabbing and eating the prey.

Orca and other dolphin calves are bonded with their mothers, yet independent. All of the skills young dolphins learn while their parents watch and keep them safe help them grow up to be functioning members of their pod. No thirty-year-old dolphins end up back in their childhood room, eating pizza their mom ordered, and lacking in motivation.

Gently nudging, role modeling, supporting, guiding, and encouraging self-reliance and independence are powerful tools parents can use to help their children develop self-motivation towards health, happiness, and success. In fact, studies show that when parents stay engaged throughout their children's young adult years with a consistent but decreasingly firm hand, their children generally do much better in life.[1] This is exactly what dolphin parents do and human parents should be doing more so—but, of course, this is easier said than done. However, if dolphins can do it, so can we!

Bonding, Role Modeling, and Guiding

The dolphin parent's main parenting tools are bonding, role modeling, and guiding. Every parent loves their child, but not every parent is bonded to their child. Being *bonded* means really knowing your child for who he is, not who you want your child to be. It's about accepting your child despite what you may see, loving her and connecting with her not just as your child, but as an individual.

Role modeling is about showing who you are on the inside *through* what you do on the outside. Children know when a mismatch exists between the two, so don't even bother preaching something you don't really believe—you'll be seen as a hypocrite, and it will likely backfire. For example, I have a hard time with remembering things such as my cellphone, keys, wallet, and often my entire purse! My children know it, so when they lose something, I'm in no position to give them a lecture about remembering their belongings. What I do tell them is that forgetting things causes stress in my life. I tell them I'm working towards being better at remembering, and if they have any ideas to help me, to let me know! So role modeling is about using your genuine self to teach life lessons, and those lessons can certainly be found in things we're good at or not so good at.

Guiding is being in a place of knowledge and/or authority, while also respecting autonomy. Parents who guide provide a tour of the world and point out life's ups and downs for their children while still providing information and support along the way. They say things like, "hey, this is where life can be unfair," "these are the ways people resolve conflict," and "this is a beautiful moment to celebrate." However, guiding parents don't complete the journey for their child—they have their own journeys.

Shoulder to Shoulder versus Face-to-Face

If a parent fully occupies the control center of a child's life, no room is left for the child to join in and make his or her own choices. In order to encourage children to develop their independence, parents must give up some control. There is simply no other way to do it.

Think about children's progress through physical development—from being immobile to mobile. Children start life fully dependent on us physically, and we literally have to carry them around. Naturally and with adequate nurturing, they gradually become more physically independent, but for many years they still need us to pick them up when they fall down or are tired. Sometimes, we still have to wipe their noses when they're sick, but in general most parents don't stand in the way of physical growth and independence. We accept the physical awkwardness and clumsiness of preteens and adolescents as a given, and we hope to stand shoulder to shoulder with them eventually, or even have them tower over us. We accept that they occupy their own physical space, and we definitely don't want to carry them around as adults.

Dolphin parents accept the principles of mental growth and independence. They provide children with a safe environment in which to fall and be clumsy in their decisions, and they pick them up or help wipe away their mess when they're young. They encourage independence as soon as possible. As children grow older, they guide them to get up on their own and clean up their own mess. They don't fully control their children's lives. They increasingly move from face-to-face authority (for example, "I know what's best for you") to shoulder-to-shoulder guide (for example, "You know what's best for you, but I'm always here to help"). In doing so, they strive to stand beside their children—independent, yet connected. Dolphin parents are happy to see their children develop their own ideas and talents, and sometimes they even tolerate opinions that may differ from their own! When parents encourage independence, children show more self-reliance, better problem solving, and improved emotional health.[2]

The first step of the dolphin way is to acknowledge to your children (and yourself) that ultimately they're in control and responsible for their own mind, body, and life. At the same time, it's important to state that you'll remain a source of guidance and support for them whenever they need you.

Dolphin parenting involves two separate processes. The first, which is highly effective on its own, is to shake off the tiger behaviors that stand in the way of what parents want to accomplish. The second is to add in specific dolphin behaviors that enhance internal control and self-motivation, and lead to independence.

Prescription

Shake Off the Authoritarian Tiger

Tigers don't allow their children to develop an internal locus of control and thus squash self-motivation and CQ. Keeping that in mind, stop overdoing the following:

- **Pushing** ("Your dad and I expect you to keep playing the piano under all circumstances …")
- **Directing/instructing** ("These are the courses you should take in grade eleven …")
- **Hovering** ("What is that spelling mistake on your homework? Did you tell your coach you want more time to play? I will help with whatever you need until you get into college …")
- **Rescuing or solving all their problems** ("You were having trouble with your best friend, so I met with her mother and it's all sorted out …")
- **Doing things your children can do for themselves** ("I made photocopies of your group homework assignment …")
- **Adding pressure for short-term performance** ("It's really important that you win the junior school dance recital …")
- **Setting goals for your children without their input** ("We invited Chelsea over so that the two of you can be friends …")

Notice I said stop *overdoing* not stop *doing* the above. We shouldn't fall into the trap of "all or nothing" thinking. Dolphin parenting doesn't mean *no* hovering and *no* directing. Of course, especially in the early years, we must direct and hover over our children for certain things—such as eating fruits and vegetables, washing hands, doing math, and reading.

Remember—dolphins are definitely *not* permissive jellyfish parents, providing no rules and no guidance. Dolphin parents are balanced and have rules and the highest expectations, but they still encourage internal control and independence in their children. They maintain authority but are not authoritarian.

PRESCRIPTION

Use Statements and Behaviors That Foster Your Child's Internal Control

When my five-year-old was complaining about going to kindergarten, it wasn't easy to tell him, "I can make you go to school now, but I can't make you listen when you get there. I can't make you learn or have fun. Only you can do those things for yourself." However, as the words were flowing out of my mouth, I could see his anxiety settle down and his anger at me dissipate. I could see the mix of uncertainty and confidence on his face as he heard the responsibility of his education being squarely placed on his shoulders, not mine.

You can never make too many statements of personal control to your child—and especially to a teenager. No matter how much we want to believe it or wish it weren't true, *nobody* likes to be told what to do, including children of well-meaning, highly intelligent, and loving parents. Resistance occurs when anyone feels their personal freedom is being controlled or threatened. The deep desire to hold autonomy over our own lives through choice is just a truth about human nature—something all of us, including our children, feel.

However, I'm not advocating for you to say to your children, "It's your life, do what you want." I'm also not saying that you should let your children make all kinds of life-changing mistakes. I'm suggesting that you gradually move shoulder to shoulder with your children as they develop their autonomy, all the while acknowledging that you're their role model and guide—not the controller of their lives.

Dolphin parents of young children may say things like, "Although I can make you go to school now, I won't be able to do that forever—it will ultimately be your choice"; "I expect you to give piano a good try, but I can't force you to like it"; "Even though I think being honest is really important, it's up to you to decide for yourself if that's true"; or "I may be able to make you do your homework right now, but I can't make you appreciate why it's important. That's something you'll have to decide on your own."

Dolphin parents of older children may say things like, "I can't control how you think or feel—how you react to the world is your choice"; "I can only guide you to do the right thing now, but what you do in your future is up to you"; "Everyone wants control of their choices—including you"; or "I can't control how your mind works so in the end it's up to you how hard you will try."

However, let's be clear, consequences do arise when you give up some external control over your children. When you say that you can only give advice but that your children must decide what to do with that advice, you need to be prepared to accept your children's decisions. And, yes, sometimes that means letting them make mistakes right in front of your eyes, which is the hardest, kick-in-the-stomach feeling for any parent. However, knowing that you'll be there to help them if and when they fall will certainly help get rid of that feeling.

PRESCRIPTION

Ask Permission Before Giving Advice

Many children and almost all teenagers are resistant to advice and suggestions, even if they're "for your own good!" Ask your children whether they would welcome your input before you give it and, trust me, things will go *much* smoother. My husband coaches soccer and says that a coach's first task is just to sit back and watch everyone's natural ability. He read one of my papers on motivation and started asking each player (and their parents) if they wanted to know what he had observed—which skills were going well, and which weren't going well. Just by asking for permission before giving advice, he was able to build an alliance with the players and their families, moving from face-to-face to shoulder-to-shoulder relationships. This simple gesture does wonders for his personal connection with players, and he finds everyone far more motivated to follow advice and suggestions.

Anthony was thirteen and having trouble with some of his friends. They were picking on him and making him the butt of all their jokes. The more his mom would tell him to "stand up for himself," the more he stood up for his friends and defended them. Anthony's mom believed in him, and told him that he "deserved better." However, that seemed to drive Anthony closer towards his friends and farther from her. One day, Anthony's friends posted an unflattering Facebook picture of his acne. This time, his mom didn't say a word. She noticed that Anthony was upset and said, "Anthony, sweetheart, tell me if you want to know what I would do in this situation." This question opened the door for Anthony to be less defensive, and he eventually asked for his mom's advice.

Once you have permission to give advice, how do you have a fruitful conversation? Try asking open-ended questions and changing the speaking/listening ratio.

PRESCRIPTION

Ask Open-Ended Questions

Open-ended questions help you express empathy and avoid arguments. They also go a long way in terms of finding out what's really going on with your child or teenager. For example, when I asked my son the closed-ended question, "Why did you skip soccer practice?" he answered, "I didn't want to go." Not much information there. But when I followed up with a question in an open-ended way, "What happened in your day today?" my son said, "Joey punched me in the back for no reason, and I was so tired after school that I didn't want to go to practice." I immediately went from being annoyed and wanting to start an argument to being empathic and concerned. Open-ended questions also foster children's independence by allowing them to determine which way the conversation will go. When you're helping your child with a homework problem, asking, "What do you think about that question?" versus "What is the answer?" or openly asking, "What would happen if you tried it a different way?" versus "Try it this way" encourages independent thinking and problem solving.

Kam found that every time she tried to talk to her daughter, Rubi, her daughter would shut down, look at the floor, and mutter, "I don't know." I coached Kam in approaching things differently. I asked her first to ask permission before launching into a discussion: "Hey Rubi, is this a good time to talk?" was one thing she could ask her daughter. She then tried asking open-ended questions such as "What's on your mind?" "How's school going?" or "Anything new with your friends?" These questions would provide Rubi with the opportunity to direct the conversation towards what was important to her. Kam tried to resist the urge to start correcting and problem solving for Rubi. I made her practice saying "Oh, that's interesting, tell me more ..." when she really wanted to say "You should do this ..." or even "What are you going to do about it?" By asking open-ended questions, Kam was able to prove to Rubi that she didn't always have an agenda and that she didn't want to engage in conversation just to "catch" her at something or "fix" something. Kam's questions showed that she was just genuinely interested in Rubi's life. They also provided space for Rubi to take on her own problem solving and become more independent. It wasn't easy for Kam to see Rubi struggle with certain issues, and it was pure torture when Rubi made a decision that made no sense or one that Kam knew would backfire. However, unless the decision was going to lead to some irreversible damage for Rubi, Kam learned to hold back and stay out of the way of the natural clumsiness that's part of growing up. Kam felt reassured knowing that she would help if and when it became critical to step in. I told Kam that it's better to be clumsy when you're fifteen and living at home than when you're twenty-four and on your own.

PRESCRIPTION

Change the Speaking/Listening Ratio

Often parents say to their children, "let's talk," and then end up doing around 80 percent of the talking. This turns a conversation into a lecture. Neurons in our brains connect around ideas a person *speaks* more than around those a person *hears*. Flip the 80:20 parent–child speaking ratio on its head. At least aim for a 70:30 ratio in which your child talks 70 percent of the time, while you listen and limit your own speaking to only 30 percent of the time, if that. It means that instead of lecturing about the problems associated with drinking alcohol, ask your child how she would explain to a younger sibling or friend or neighbor the problems associated with drinking. It means instead of talking about how important homework is, ask your child to tell you why it might be important to him or her. This technique may get your child to say what you are dying to say!

Trudy found that her talks quickly turned into shouting matches with her twelve-year-old son, Max. She decided to change the speaking/listening ratio and simply held back on how much she was interrupting Max and speaking herself. Just by talking less, she found that Max would practically talk himself out of his own argument! For example, Max said that he didn't want to do his homework one night. Instead of launching into a 70:30 parent–child lecture on how important homework is, she simply said, "What's going on?" Max explained that he didn't like his teacher because she gave too much homework. If he didn't do it, she would give even more, and he was going to get a low grade, which was unfair. He then said the homework wasn't even that hard and was a waste of time. When he got no reaction from his mom, other than "You're right, that sounds unfair, but what are your other options?" Max ran out of things to say and lost steam for his argument. He procrastinated a bit and eventually did his homework.

PRESCRIPTION

Review Benefits and Drawbacks

Discussing a behavior's benefits and drawbacks is a great open-ended way to get your child thinking (and speaking) about not only the positive but also the negative aspects of a behavior. If you want your discussions to go well, it's important for you to be open to talking about issues your child may not expect you to be open about. Take the issue of drinking. You have come to terms with the idea that your teenager may be drinking behind your back at parties. You've expressed your clear desire for him to not let it get out of hand. Surprise him by asking him to tell you about all the benefits he sees with drinking at a party. Maybe he believes that drinking offers physical benefits, such as feeling more energetic for dancing, or perhaps psychological benefits, such as feeling less self-conscious around girls. Then ask him about the downsides of drinking at a party, and you'll be surprised at how much your child has to say. This type of discussion is the first step towards really understanding what's going on in your child's mind; and it's only by understanding that we can be an effective guide.

PRESCRIPTION

Rate Benefits and Drawbacks

After reviewing a behavior's benefits and drawbacks, ask your child to rank each benefit and drawback on a scale from one to ten, with one being the least important to them and ten being the most important. Let's say your child is having a hard time balancing Facebook time and exercise. One benefit of Facebook time might be connecting with friends—a possible ten for your child. One drawback is that too much time spent on Facebook may get parents angry—a possible seven for your child. However, worse drawbacks might be, "I get caught up in all the drama and usually message something I regret"—which is likely a ten—and "I then get upset, eat too much, and feel gross." The ten is where you will find the child's self-motivation towards positive change. If you know where the motivation lies, you can help your child problem solve to find other ways of connecting with friends without the downsides—and freeing up some more time for exercise!

PRESCRIPTION

Use Statements and Behaviors That Emphasize Commitment and Support for Your Child

Despite the emphasis on personal control, dolphin parents make it clear that they're fully committed and available to their child for support and guidance. The children of dolphin parents know that they're a priority in their parents' lives and that their parents will "always be there" when needed. Dolphin parents make statements like, "I will always be there for you"; "If you need me, I will come"; "I will still love you no matter what"; and "You can always ask for my advice or help." Dolphin parents make good on their promises and are there to support and encourage their children during those times of need. In doing so, they're also enhancing their bonding as well as role modeling what it means to be in a loving, supportive relationship. Although these statements and behaviors may seem natural for parents, they're not self-evident. I've heard many tiger parents express conditional love for their children; for example, "Mommy will spend some time with you as soon as you play violin in the conservatory."

PRESCRIPTION

To Motivate, Focus on Importance and Confidence

Now all of this is fine, but how do you get your child to get to school on time or finish their homework when they're whining? Importance and confidence are strong motivators for action. When a task has *importance*, a person understands "what's in it for me" or the reasons why the task is necessary. When a person has *confidence*, that person believes that she can accomplish the task. A task must meet these two criteria for a child (or anyone) to want to act.

Explain (or Find Out) Why a Task Is Important

Knowing why a task is important clearly helps build motivation for it. In a Harvard study, participants were divided into two groups and asked to build LEGO Bionicles characters. All participants were paid for their work in decreasing amounts: $3 for the first one, $2.70 for the next one, etc. One group's characters were stored and then disassembled at the end of the experiment. The other group's characters were disassembled immediately after they were created, right in front of participants' eyes. On average, the group that saw their characters immediately destroyed made five characters less than the other group before quitting, even though they were getting paid the same amount as the other group for their work. For me, this experiment points to two conclusions: money alone is not enough of a motivator, even for something as neutral as building LEGO chacters, and that a task without "meaning" or "importance" quickly derails motivation.[3]

Explaining rules is a consistent feature in balanced parenting styles across cultures. Research shows that by simply explaining the reason behind the rule, children become more "empathic, helpful, conscientious, and kind to others."[4]

Whether it's math, piano, or homework, children don't want to do something just because they're told to do it. Make sure children understand why they're doing what they're doing (make sure you know why too!). Just because you think a task is important, that doesn't mean your child does. Children have no idea why fruits and vegetables are "good" for them and why cotton candy is not. They really have no reason to believe homework is important unless the lessons behind the tasks are explained. That explanation can even be as basic as "practice makes you better at something, so all you are doing now is practicing math." Look for and point out reasons the task is important for your child. For younger children, link short-term importance with long-term importance. Because they may have a hard time fully understanding long-term consequences, always look for what is important to them—not you. For example, my son had no idea why he had to take French in school and opposed it strongly (it is part of the Canadian curriculum). When I gave him all *my* reasons—such as "French is a great language," "it's good for your brain development," and "maybe it will help you get a job one day"—he didn't disagree, but it didn't help get him to practice his French any better. Once I told him that knowing French would make it easier for him to learn Spanish, he suddenly showed more interest and motivation. You see, my son (who is eight) dreams of playing soccer for FC Barcelona one day, "just like Lionel Messi," so now he's even motivated to learn Spanish!

Understand Your Child's Confidence Level

Confidence is half the equation when it comes to motivation, and we rarely ask about it. For example, many doctors spend a lot of time telling their patients that smoking causes lung cancer and emphysema, yet how many smokers nowadays don't know this fact? In this case, it's not the importance that's the problem, it's the confidence. If they could "wish upon a star," most adults would probably rank the level of importance of quitting smoking high, but rank their level of confidence in quitting low. What we doctors really need to do is discuss how to improve confidence rather than focus on importance.

In my experience, when it comes to low motivation for things that are generally considered positive—quitting smoking, going to school, exercising, getting along better with others—the issue is confidence, not importance. For example, most high school students know the importance of a high school diploma. They know you need it for any job, including a Starbucks barista job (for which you may even need a degree now). However, confidence to get that diploma is not necessarily a given, especially for a child with a learning disability or attention deficit hyperactivity disorder (ADHD), which can make academics even harder. Children often get endless lectures about how important school is, but most of them already know that—the issue is confidence.

Bring Importance and Confidence Together

The importance and confidence scale can help you determine your child's view of the importance of a task and his or her confidence level in the ability to undertake that task.

Let's say your child is showing resistance to or ambivalence about a task, such as graduating high school. Consider asking the following two questions about it:[5]

- **Question 1 (on importance):** On a scale of one to ten, with ten being very important, how important is it for you to graduate high school?
- **Question 2 (on confidence):** On that same scale, how confident are you that you can graduate high school?

By asking about a task's importance and confidence rankings, the real issue holding back your child will come out. It's then that you can address it.

Let's say your child is lacking motivation to prepare for a test. You might ask: "On a scale of one to ten, with ten being very important, how important is this test for you?" If your child says, "Well, I think it's irrelevant for my life, but I want to graduate with all my friends, so I guess it's an eight," then you might ask, "OK, on the same scale, how confident are you that you can get the grade you want?" Your child might respond, "That's a three. My teacher is so unfair; no matter how hard I try, I just can't seem to do well." Clearly, the issue here is the child's confidence, and that means that no amount of lecturing about the importance of the test will enhance the child's self-motivation to do well. Instead, you would need to work with your child to help problem solve the issue with the teacher and restore the child's confidence.

PRESCRIPTION

Use the Dolphin KEYS to Motivate

Knowing that both importance and confidence are needed for motivation, how can we motivate children to do everyday tasks without them driving us parents nuts! Of course, communication is essential, but not just any communication. Our children are highly attuned to our tone of voice, stance, facial expression, and all other non-verbal cues. So, what we say and how we say it are important. I developed a four-step process for effective motivational communication—called the *dolphin KEYS*—which I've been using for over ten years. This process may not work the first time, and you may need some practice to get it right, but its cumulative effects are helpful for motivating your child.

The four steps that make up the dolphin KEYS are the essence of motivational communication. They complement but don't intrude on your child's development of his or her self-motivation. The four steps have been adapted from the four basic principles of motivational interviewing—a therapy proven to enhance motivation—developed by professors Bill Miller (University of New Mexico) and Steve Rollnick (University of Cardiff).[6] If you follow these four steps, all communication will be more effective and easier.

> **Step 1: Kill the tiger.** If the tiger is roaring within you, start with a few deep, controlled breaths and make sure you're calm before you proceed.
>
> **Step 2: Empathize.** Express that you understand your child and that you are on his or her side.
>
> **Step 3: Identify Your child's goals.** You are now in your child's shoes, so acknowledge his or her goals (rather than focusing on your own goals).
>
> **Step 4: Support success.** Express belief in your child's ability to carry out the task.

Step 1: Kill the tiger. Being an angry, roaring tiger simply doesn't work. Behavioral science tells us that arguing is highly counterproductive, especially if the goal is to convince someone to change a certain behavior. In fact, it's been shown that the process of arguing tends to entrench a person further in his or her own beliefs.[7] I demonstrate this all the time in my workshops. I ask participants to pair off. Then each person tries to convince his or her partner that the ocean is either blue or green. It's no surprise that after about three minutes, each person only further believes in his or her own position.

With children, resistance is a signal to change strategies. As we all know, the more you push children (or anyone for that matter), the more they resist, which often makes them more (outwardly or internally) defiant. This is especially true for teenagers.

So, if you find yourself in a yelling match with your child, and the child is defending a position you don't want to further entrench—for example, that "marijuana is not that bad"—*stop*, do something else, and come back to the issue at a later time without the argument. I know this sounds impossible when you're revved up with adrenaline about a particular issue. However, that's why you must leave the situation, take a few breaths, calm down, and re-center. Once the tiger is out of your way, you can create an environment of balance and guidance.

Step 2: Empathize. Empathy has long been a powerful tool for human bonding and motivation. Empathy is not sympathy. *Empathy* is the ability to "walk a mile in another's shoes," to really understand what another is going through, to sit *within* the experience. In contrast, *sympathy* is the ability to express sorrow for someone's situation, to sit *with* the experience.

Empathy is not to be taken lightly. It's exceedingly powerful yet constantly overlooked or disregarded. It's the basis of any relationship and becomes especially important if things get off track. In over a decade of working with children and teenagers, I've seen firsthand that empathy is often the only thing that can help improve a situation. Everyone wants to be listened to, and everyone believes their opinions and ideas count. Everyone wants to be understood and, most of all, everyone wants to be loved and accepted unconditionally.

Children don't want to be loved and accepted only when they're on their good behavior or compliant with external expectations. Thus, displays of empathy are particularly critical when things aren't going well or a relationship is strained. Empathy doesn't equate with approval of a problem behavior, but it does signal your effort to understand the feelings and possible reasons behind it. Empathy shows acceptance for who your child is—weaknesses and all. For example, parents can fully disapprove of their child's use of marijuana, but still "accept" their child.

Expressing empathy to your child builds an alliance with him or her. That alliance makes it more likely that your child will turn to you for help now and in the future. Most important, acceptance facilitates change. Only when children feel fully accepted for who they are will they be more likely to change. Otherwise, they'll be entrenched in proving that who they are deserves acceptance. A young person who smokes marijuana will be resentful and unlikely to change if he feels acceptance and love are contingent upon quitting.

Empathy also helps improve your child's self-esteem, particularly because chances are good that she may be feeling alone in her difficulties or blaming herself. Since we were all children once, letting your child know that you made mistakes too or had the same feelings when you were young is a great way to express empathy.

Empathic statements include:

- "Help me understand what you're thinking/feeling."
- "I can see you don't want to do your homework right now."
- "I can see you're really upset."
- "I can appreciate this is really hard for you."
- "I wish you could play too."
- "I don't want to break up all the fun, however …"

Step 3: Identify your child's goals. People do things for a reason, and their behavior is motivated by personal values and goals. The same is true for children. Of course, sometimes it's necessary to use external control by threats and rewards to influence behavior, and I use these in my own parenting at times (for example, while writing this page, I told my son that we would return his gecko to the store if he didn't clean his tank). However, the resulting behavior may not last beyond the immediate, so the sooner a parent starts encouraging personal internal control, the better.

For children to internalize motivation, they need to connect behavior with their own goals. Try to help your child understand how current behavior may positively or negatively affect his or her personal goals. When your child is acting out, point out the discrepancy between the behavior and the goals your child has expressed. You might suggest that acting in a way contrary to those goals may get in the way of achieving what he or she hopes to achieve.

If the connection between your children's behavior and their goals is unclear, it's far more effective if children themselves, not parents, make the connection. However, parents can certainly guide their children to make that connection. Have a look at the following two scenarios. By expressing empathy and identifying the connection between behavior and goals, the parent is guiding the child to solve her own problems, and the child says what she truly wants to say.

Scenario 1:

PARENT. What do you think will happen if you keep demanding that I give you this cookie? [asked calmly and with empathy]

CHILD. I don't know. You'll give it to me?

PARENT. No, in fact, if you're rude and pushy, it will make me *not* want to give it to you. Do you have any ideas that may help you get what you want?

CHILD. I could ask nicely.

PARENT. Yes, what else?

CHILD. I could be patient and wait for you to finish what you're doing.

Scenario 2:

PARENT. What do you think will happen to your basketball playing if you keep skipping your homework? [asked calmly and with empathy]

CHILD. My annoying teacher will talk to the coach, who will bench me. You said you're not going to keep taking me to basketball camp if my grades drop, so I'll likely not play enough, and then I won't make next year's team.

PARENT. So do you think doing homework will move you closer or farther away from your goal of playing basketball next year?

CHILD. Closer, I guess.

In scenarios like the two above, parents may really want to say something like, "Ask nicely!" or "If you don't smarten up with your homework, you'll be off the basketball team!" but that's less effective than when a child draws the same conclusion and says it aloud. Remember, our neurons synapse around the words we speak more than what we hear.

Step 4: Support success. People change when they believe something is important *and* when they feel they're capable of the change. Anything parents can do to support and encourage belief in the ability to change will also support and encourage that change. Children often feel they'll fall short of the expectations of their parents, so parents' hope and optimism for their children's true abilities help children feel more confident. Parents who say, "I know you're capable of understanding this," "I'm sure you'll find a solution," and "I know you'll make the right decision" are on the right track. Statements like these put the onus of responsibility squarely on the child; like the beached dolphin, the child must find his or her own way "back to open water." As you proactively try to develop your children's self-motivation, remember that it's essential for them to believe in their ability to be independent.

How to Apply Dolphin KEYS to Specific Situations

Here are some examples of how to apply the dolphin KEYS to different situations. I've assumed that you've already completed step one and killed the tiger, so you'll notice the tiger is absent from the statements below, which are meant to be said without roaring!

- **Your child is late in the morning.** "I know it's hard to get going in the morning [empathize], but your goal was not to be late again [identify your child's goals]. Come on, I know you can move a little faster [support success]."
- **Your child doesn't want to do homework.** "I used to hate doing homework, too [empathize], but you don't want to miss out on free time or recess during class, [identify your child's goals]. Thank goodness you pick up things easily once you put your mind to it [support success]."
- **Your child resists going to soccer practice.** "Aw, you look so tired today [empathize], but this is the only way to prepare for that upcoming game [identify your child's goals]. You always feel great once you're on the field [support success]."
- **Your child doesn't want to practice piano.** "You're getting super frustrated and tired [empathize]. But if you don't get this song

right, you won't make it into the recital [identify your child's goals]. I know you can try just one more time [support success]."

- **Your child doesn't want to eat dinner.** "Yes, it's hard to eat food you don't like very much [empathize], but if you don't eat, we don't get to go to the park [identify your child's goals]. You did it before, so I'm sure you can do it again [support success]."

Now that we have a few prescriptions for behaviors that support dolphin parenting, let's consider what children need to *do* for health, happiness, self-motivation, and all aspects of success!

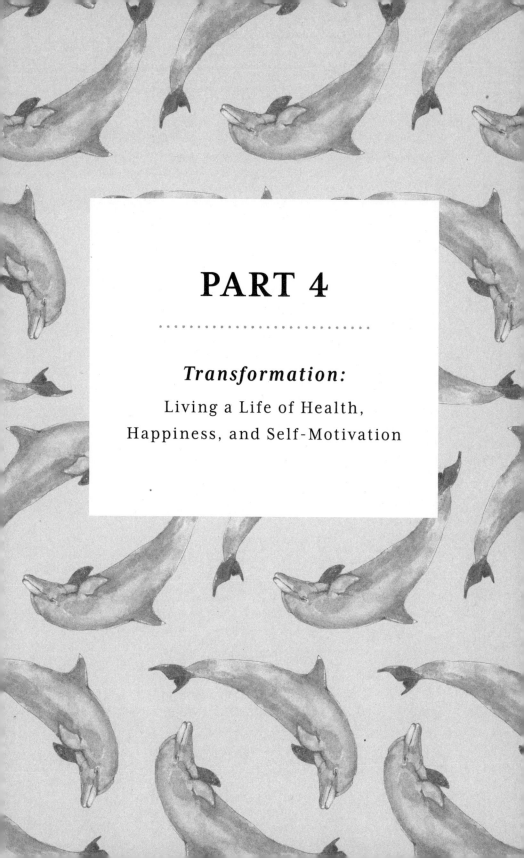

PART 4

. . . .

Transformation:

Living a Life of Health,
Happiness, and Self-Motivation

Chapter 9
. . . .

SELF-MOTIVATION IS LASTING

A glance at an early report card for Nobel prizewinner Sir John Gurdon would have been enough to convince most people that the young man was not destined for a career in science. Ranked last out of 250 biology students in his year when he was fifteen, Gurdon nevertheless expressed a desire to study science in university, which clearly exasperated his biology teacher, who was more than happy to write the following in his report card:

> I believe [Gurdon] has ideas about becoming a scientist;
> on his present showing this is quite ridiculous; If he can't
> learn simple Biological facts he would have no chance of
> doing the work of a Specialist, and it would be a sheer
> waste of time, both on his part and of those who would
> have to teach him.[1]

Gurdon went on to study Latin and Greek at Oxford, which, to many people, might seem far from a terrible fate. However, Gurdon wasn't satisfied. He still had a strong passion for science, so his parents found him a private science tutor. We all know how hard it can be for a child to catch up after missing some school, and Gurdon had a lot of ground to cover. He got down to work, and did his best to make up for lost time.

It turns out that Gurdon wasn't so terrible at science after all. He ended up completing his doctorate in zoology, and went on to revolutionize the field of cellular biology. He was made a Fellow of the Royal Society in 1971 and was knighted in 1995. In 2004, the Wellcome Trust/Cancer Research UK Institute for Cell Biology and Cancer was renamed the Gurdon Institute in his honor. He won the Nobel Prize for Physiology and Medicine in 2012 for his groundbreaking research showing that mature cells can be converted into stem cells. He had the report card from his biology teacher framed.

Fortunately for Gurdon, his curiosity fueled a self-motivation that was so strong even the toughest of tigers couldn't crush it. His CQ was so developed that he triumphed in a system that could have easily stood in the way of his Nobel-worthy mind.

If you have self-motivation, you're far less likely to fear struggle, mistakes, and failure. You're also far more likely to crave healthy doses of unstructured learning, play, and exploration. Self-motivation will help you maintain your drive through whatever struggles you must face. It will also help you take on complex cognitive and emotional challenges because you're able to think critically, be creative, communicate, and collaborate. A healthy self-motivation works synergistically with a high CQ.

We all want our children to be strong enough to deal with the obstacles they'll have to overcome in life, but are we helping them develop the kind of motivation they'll need to keep going when times are tough? None of us is going to answer no, so let's start with a different question. It may seem simple, but trust me—it's not. Do you want a compliant child or an engaged child with self-motivation? Take a moment before you answer my question.

Your answer may be that you want your child to do exactly what you tell her to. But don't you ultimately want her to take responsibility for herself and find her own path? No parents want their children living with them at thirty, with no driving curiosity, no passion, and no interest to do or be something. If you want healthy, happy, and successful children that can make it on their own, you have no choice but to nurture (and not interfere with) your child's natural self-motivation.

In contrast, your answer may be that you want an engaged child who can think for herself. (That's what I want too, by the way.) I should warn you: parenting a young person capable of independent, critical thought is much tougher than raising a compliant tiger. However, it's a lot more satisfying.

Regardless of what we want, children need self-motivation to look after themselves, whether it's cleaning up their room without having to be nagged or moving out before they turn forty.

What Is Self-Motivation?

Self-motivation is the holy grail of parenting. In fact, I would go so far as to say that it's the holy grail of all human happiness. As a doctor, I can't exaggerate how important it is. As a mother, I can't exaggerate how hard I work to instill it. Now, the fact that I have to work hard should give you a hint. Helping your child develop self-motivation is simple, but not easy.

Self-motivation "involves engaging in a behavior because it is personally rewarding."[2] Self-motivation is different from desire. For example, many of today's youth want money and status but they aren't always internally driven to work for these things. Self-motivation is wanting something enough to act on it.

Because external motivation is based on someone else's wants and not your own, action based on it will last only as long as the external pressure, demands, rewards, or punishments are in place.

Self-Motivation Is Different for Everyone

We know that our children aren't going to get far without the proper motivation. But what *is* it that drives them? One thing that makes life difficult for parents and children is that everyone views self-motivation differently. Your child may think he is totally motivated to do something, and you may think he is *not* motivated at all.

Let's say two people live three blocks away from their fitness club. Person A drives to the club and Person B walks. Do you think these two people have the same self-motivation to exercise?

Some of you will say, "No way! If Person A were serious about fitness, he would have walked to the club!" Others may say, "Both are going to the club! Who cares how they got there?" Both of these opinions are valid. Persons A and B might both be lazy bones who come to the fitness club to socialize and may hardly get a workout. Person A might be running a marathon the next day and trying to preserve energy by driving to the club. Or maybe the scenario is altogether different.

The Stages of Change

Self-motivation isn't a fixed trait—something we either have or don't have. Instead, it's dynamic and dependent on a variety of factors. Let's not pigeonhole children (or ourselves) into the "motivated" and "unmotivated" categories. Because the human brain has neuroplasticity, we can change ourselves and our behavior in wonderful and dynamic ways.

How can we help foster our children's motivation for healthy behaviors? Individuals go through a series of stages before they change behavior. Knowing which stage your child is in can help you understand their state of mind so that you can provide the appropriate support for them to succeed in making healthy changes. The six stages of change and associated support techniques are as follows:[3]

- *Precontemplation:* Individuals have no intent to change their behavior. They may be in denial or see no need for change. *Support techniques:* Validate their feelings and encourage them to evaluate their behavior. With them, list the pros and cons related to the current behavior (with empathy not judgment). Doing so can be very helpful in this stage.

- *Contemplation:* Individuals are willing to consider that their behavior might benefit from change, but they're also conflicted over reasons to change and not to change. *Support techniques:* Encourage them to think about the advantages and disadvantages of changing their behavior, and bring to their attention the positive outcomes of the behavior change.

- *Determination/preparation:* Individuals begin to see that the advantages of changing their behavior are greater than the advantages of continuing with their current behavior. They're ready for and committed to taking action but have not made any concrete steps towards change yet. *Support techniques:* Examine obstacles to change, and help them problem solve; identify the support they can rely on during the change; and suggest that they take small initial steps.

- *Action:* Individuals believe that they can change their behavior and begin to actively do so. Individuals rely on their self-motivation to stay in action. "People in this stage also tend to be open to receiving help and are also likely to seek support from others (a very important element)."[4] *Support techniques:* Reinforce their self-efficacy for handling obstacles, and remind them of the long-term benefits of the new behavior.

- *Maintenance:* Individuals in this stage try to sustain the new behavior and avoid the influences (for example, people or situations) that would lead them to fall back into the problematic behavior. They tend to remind themselves of the good progress they've made. *Support techniques:* Reinforce the internal rewards that the new change has provided.

- *Relapse/recycle:* At some point, self-motivation may wane (remember, it can fluctuate) and individuals might return to their problematic behavior. *Support techniques:* At this point, it's helpful to evaluate with the individual what triggered the relapse and plan coping strategies or barriers to those triggers that can lead the individual to get back on track.

Let's walk through these stages with the case of homework. In the precontemplation stage, your child may be thinking: *Homework? Not for me. I'm passing everything I need to. I'm going on Facebook.* Then comes contemplation: *I really want to get on Facebook, but I should do my homework or I may fail that class.* After a while, determination/preparation sets in, usually based on new information: *I failed the last assignment. I'll fail the class if I don't start paying attention to my homework.* Next come action and maintenance, maybe in the form of a whole month of doing homework on time with no troubles, and then ... relapse: *The teacher hates me anyway. I don't find the subject interesting, and there's no chance of passing. Forget homework. Back to Facebook.*

Movement through these different stages is natural. No one—and especially not children—can be in the stage of action for every activity or behavior all the time. Despite that truth, many parents expect their children to be in the action stage for the activities and behaviors they (the parents) consider important. I've had parents come and ask me if their child has attention deficit disorder (ADD) because that child "can't seem to focus" in school. As I take the child's history, I find out that the child's schedule is packed solid from morning to night with school, after-school activities, and then homework. How can anyone sustain attention with a schedule like that? The majority of children don't lack motivation at all. If your child can't sustain straight As, competitive sports, competitive music, and no downtime, all that means is that your child's perfectly normal! To develop self-motivation for any behavior, we need to be able to move from one stage of change to the next with some level of energy.

A Life of Balance: The Basis for Self-Motivation

Consider self-motivation as part of a hierarchy of motivation. Of course, we're first driven towards the basics of survival—covered in Chapter 5—including nourishment and sleep. We can all relate to being unmotivated and sluggish when we're hungry, thirsty, or sleepy. And we know that humans are biologically hardwired to play, explore, bond socially, and contribute as well. These activities are also essential to our survival as a species, and we're thus internally motivated and rewarded by engaging in them. Once we've achieved some kind of balance in these fundamentals, we gain vitality and some drive towards continuous challenge. If you think about people around you who have vitality, you'll notice that they also have self-motivation. Vitality requires the basic ingredients of survival and a balance among all of them. More of one of these basics doesn't lead a person to be more motivated (for example, eating healthy food or drinking water beyond the amount we need to feel well-nourished doesn't improve motivation).

We're biologically motivated to find a balance among our survival activities. For example, a sleep-deprived child will be motivated to sleep; and if that child continues to be sleep deprived, she will become dysregulated and insomnia will settle in. The same is true for a child who is deprived of play or social bonds; he will be motivated to fulfill these needs before "work." In addition, we know that young brains are more rewarded for some activities and thus more motivated to do them. For young children, it's sleeping and playing; and for adolescents, it's social bonding and exploring. Children are always going to be motivated—the question is which motivation is going to prevail. So, in many ways, parenting is "motivation management."

Curiosity: The Foundation for Self-motivation

Eleanor Roosevelt once said, "I think, at a child's birth, if a mother could ask a fairy godmother to endow it with the most useful gift, that gift should be curiosity."[5]

When we're balanced, curiosity—a key factor in self-motivation—can flourish. Humans (and dolphins) are driven by natural curiosity, the desire for knowledge. Without it, we wouldn't have the motivation to explore the world around us. It should come as no surprise that curiosity is linked to our brain's dopamine reward system. Curiosity is hardwired into our brains and is the fuel that keeps the self-motivation for learning going.

Despite our vast knowledge of the brain, we actually know little about curiosity. In a recent Caltech study, undergraduate students were asked to answer forty trivia questions while they were in a brain scanner.[6] After reading each question, the subjects were told to silently guess the answer and to indicate their curiosity about the correct answer. Then, they were presented with the question again, along with the correct answer. During this experiment, scientists found that several key parts of the brain were stimulated more than others when the students indicated their curiosity: the prefrontal cortex (the thinking part of the brain), the parahippocampal gyrus (where memories are encoded and retrieved), and the caudate. The caudate has long been associated with knowledge and learning and, more recently, emotion. In fact, it may be the caudate that connects new knowledge with strong and powerful positive emotions, such as love. To me, this is a perfect description of curiosity. When we fall in love with what we're curious about, it becomes our "passion." And passion is certainly a powerful driver of motivation.[7] Curiosity leads us to "walk along" unknown neural tracks and uncover the awesome power of the human mind. Consider Albert Einstein's interesting comment: "I have no special talents, I am just passionately curious."[8]

Curiosity also calms us down. When we look at the world through curious eyes, we don't judge or react but simply observe and interact. Curiosity takes us out of fear mode and engages our thinking brain. Curiosity requires time to pause and think (imagine trying to be curious on a schedule). If you're too busy to be curious, you're too busy to be motivated.

Autonomy, Mastery, and Purpose:
The Drivers of Lasting Self-Motivation

Studies on the psychology of motivation show that we're motivated when three criteria are fulfilled: autonomy, mastery, and purpose.[9] *Autonomy* is the desire to direct and control our own lives. It comes from internal control, and parents instill it through balanced authoritative parenting. *Mastery* is the desire to keep getting better at something that matters to us. It comes from finding and developing one's passion through play. Curiosity itself is an "inverted U-shaped drive"[10]—it piques us to overcome challenges and continually stretch ourselves towards mastery. *Purpose* is our desire to do something that matters in the world—to engage in something beyond ourselves. It comes from our desire to connect and contribute.

A University of Michigan study shows that knowing that our work helps others increases even our unconscious motivation.[11] In the study, a student who had received a scholarship from a university fundraising call center was asked to speak for ten minutes to those responsible for the fundraising about how that scholarship changed his life. A month later, the fundraisers were spending 142 percent more time on the phone than before, and revenues had increased by 171 percent. But the fundraisers denied the scholarship student's ten-minute visit had influenced them. "It was almost as if the good feelings had bypassed the callers' conscious cognitive processes and gone straight to a more subconscious source of motivation. They were more driven to succeed, even if they could not pinpoint the trigger for that drive."[12]

A Life of Balance: The Strength to Meet Challenges

People are also rewarded when they're challenged. Doesn't it feel good when we achieve something we didn't know we could? Doesn't it feel even better when we figure it out on our own and in our own unique way? Any challenge inherently has two forces: struggle and joy. Without struggle, there's no joy. By definition, challenge requires venturing into unknown territory because we can't be challenged within our comfort zone. We need to explore, struggle, challenge, and overcome stress for our survival, and that's why we naturally feel great when we get through something difficult. That's another reason parents sometimes just need to get out of Mother Nature's way.

I tell my children the following story when they look at me to solve their problems, ease their struggle, or reduce their challenge:

> A little boy was watching a butterfly struggle to get out of its cocoon. The butterfly was clearly challenged and working hard to get out until the little boy decided to "help," and ripped open the cocoon for the butterfly. To the boy's shock, the butterfly didn't fly away joyfully and freely but instead stayed exactly where it was. What the little boy didn't realize was that the butterfly needed to struggle with its cocoon to develop the muscles and coordination it needed to fly.

In a similar way, children need to struggle at times to develop the mental strength and coordination they need for independence. The boy unknowingly stifled the butterfly similarly to how we parents unwittingly stifle our children's resilience and independence by stepping in too often and too soon. Self-motivation is in each of us—Mother Nature hardwired it in our brains. Parents don't need to create it; they need to avoid derailing it and crushing it altogether.

Moreover, our kids *need* to experience some stress to make them resilient. In an interesting experiment, Mark Seery, a professor at the University of Buffalo, plunged the hands of undergraduate students into ice water. He found that students who had experienced some life adversity (such as a death or an illness in the family) actually felt less pain and could tolerate the experience better than those who reported little life adversity.[13] He concluded: "Having this history of dealing with these negative things leads people to be more likely to have a propensity for general resilience ... They are better equipped to deal with even mundane, everyday stressors."[14]

Challenges are good for us. No one is suggesting that we seek out misfortune. However, a certain amount of adversity is healthy—especially in childhood—if we want to avoid becoming a "teacup" (keeping in mind that too much can make someone a "crispie").

What we want are challenges that help us learn and grow. When we face, struggle with, and overcome a challenge, our biological payoff is the activation of dopamine pathways that make us feel good. We feel tremendous joy in a job well done, and the harder the job, the better our reward and feeling of joy. "Dopamine is the fuel that keeps people motivated to persevere and achieve a goal."[15] Scientists have linked higher levels of dopamine to forming lifelong habits. In contrast, low levels of dopamine make us apathetic. "If you do not accomplish something every day your dopamine reserves will diminish. Humans are designed to work hard and to be rewarded for their efforts biologically."[16]

Psychologist Angela Duckworth looked at children and adults who successfully dealt with stressful and challenging situations to understand the key to their success.[17] The answer was "grit." In a landmark study, she researched 2,800 subjects, from West Point Military Academy cadets, National Spelling Bee participants, salespeople, to teachers in tough neighborhoods to determine the factors that predicted their success. Grit was the consistent factor. For example, grit was a greater predictor than SAT scores, class rank, and physical fitness in determining who would survive the US military's famous West Point Academy hellish summer boot camp.

Stress, challenge, and passion are all dependent and regulated by our biology's natural feedback loop. Thus, we can't lose our balance along the path towards achievement. Have you ever accomplished something really big and noticed that the joy was either short-lived or missing? That happens when the costs of the achievement outweigh its benefits. These costs are often associated with our health and relationships. They can accumulate when we either intentionally or unintentionally neglect those things in the hot pursuit of achievement. Too often, I've heard about busy parents who spent so much time chasing receding goals like wealth and image that their children grew up at a distance. Feeling sad, empty, or "not right" is Mother Nature's way of reminding us that we're not meeting our basic needs for a balanced life. You can try to ignore, mask, or escape these feelings through more pursuit and more achievement, but you can't fool your own biology.

Being off balance, pushed into things, or having things done for us actually deprives us of the joy of overcoming a challenge and the associated feeling of well-being and joy that comes from it. That's why real-world learning that includes trial and error, and even failure, must not be seen as devastating, as it is by tiger parents. Overcoming challenges is part of life and a powerful way to learn what really matters: how to adapt.

Tigers Kill Self-Motivation

After yelling, bribing, and punishing didn't persuade my son to do his homework, one day I thought to myself, *This is unreal: I can help a drug-addicted teenager quit cocaine, but I can't get my seven-year-old to write down the alphabet!* Then it hit me: with all my experience in motivating young people to quit drinking, control their video-gaming, treat their depression, manage their anxiety, talk to their parents, break up with their no-good boyfriends, and stop abusing Adderall, I was forgetting to apply the principles that work in my practice to my own parenting. The fact is that I can't force, plead with, or command my child to be motivated to do homework any more than I can force, plead with, or command my patients to become healthy. Directing a child to do something or doing it for him doesn't work, and we all know it. Yet these practices are the essence of tiger parenting—practices that lead children to become dependent on external rewards and develop an external locus of control.

If your children master something solely because of external pressure, they'll most likely come to dislike it and eventually stop doing it—even if they have a natural talent for it. I see this all the time in my practice, and it often happens around high school. Many of those tiger cubs who were bolting out of the gates and destroying the competition as children start to plateau and are often passed over by others who may have experienced a more relaxed dolphin approach to their academic and extracurricular activities. Some don't care that they're falling behind, and some are even thankful, because they're burnt out. Others can't handle being less than the "best" and fall apart instead of trying harder because they're as fragile as a teacup. Young people who want to excel and win a competition at the high school level need CQ to do it, but they haven't developed CQ skills because they've been living in a bubble of endless activities and practice since they were toddlers.

External rewards go hand-in-hand with external motivation. When we motivate via toys, money, or too much praise, we also take away the chance for internal rewards—that amazing dose of dopamine that keeps us feeling happy.

Sam Glucksberg, a professor of psychology at Princeton University, showed just how problematic external rewards can be when it comes to self-motivation—especially for tasks that require CQ.[18] Glucksberg divided study participants into two groups and asked both of them to solve a problem requiring critical analysis as fast as possible. He told both groups they would be timed. One group was told that their time would just be used to reflect the average time it would typically take someone to solve the problem; the message was that there was no pressure to perform because the data would be used only for interest. The other group was given financial incentives: "If you're in the top 25 percent of the fastest times, you get five dollars. If you're the fastest of everyone we're testing here today, you get 20 dollars."[19] Who do you think solved the puzzle faster? The group with the money incentive or the group with no incentive? The group that was offered money actually took considerably more time—an average of three-and-a-half minutes—than the group that wasn't offered money. This study proves that motivation by reward doesn't enhance creative thinking and problem solving. In fact, it appears to dull or slow down critical thinking and creativity because of the narrow focus on the reward.

Pushing, hovering, demanding, and cajoling may get results when tasks are simple, but when tasks become complex, involve creativity, and require critical thinking, these external motivators work poorly. Sure, a child motivated by bribes and threats may reach a decent, maybe even good, level of skill in an area. For example, the more ballet a child is pushed into and given rewards for, the better ballet dancer she may become for a short period of time. But carrots and sticks can't replace autonomy, mastery, and purpose as the foundation of self-motivation. Nor can they lead to feelings of satisfaction, pleasure, and joy. Fulfilling our curiosity through our own efforts leads to satisfaction, and contributing to the greater good leads to joy. As children grow older, they must develop internal rewards over external rewards to develop self-motivation and true independence. Being great at something requires adaptability and CQ. Of course, if technical skill is all that's required to become the world's greatest at something, children that rely on external motivators may accomplish that as long as no real-life obstacles get in the way. However, more often than not, after the first major injury, jealous teammate, horrible boss, or the stress of not living under the parents' protection, things go astray for these children. In many ways, overfocusing on short-term performance and achievement gets in the way of long-term success.

At best, tiger parenting focuses on mastery alone, only if the child (not the parent) finds the activity important enough to want to master it. At worst, tiger parenting completely fails to instill self-motivation in children.

If we want our children to have self-motivation, then we must also display self-motivation. This means that we need to put an end to external motivation driven by fear. If we want to role model self-motivation, we must live a balanced lifestyle that includes play, exploration, community, and contribution. We must also take risks, step out of our comfort zones, challenge ourselves, and not let the fear of failure stop us.

Children must believe that it's OK *not* to be perfect. Let your children put on their own clothes—even if they're mismatched and backwards. Own up to your imperfections with your children. They can see them anyway, so you might as well show them that you accept yourself but are also willing to improve. My children *love* pointing out my small blunders: "Mom, you forgot your phone again!"

Mistakes are great learning experiences. Let your child screw up a homework project once in a while. That's how they'll learn what they need to do differently next time. This is easier said than done, and deep breaths certainly help. Children need to know that everyone makes mistakes, that mistakes can be corrected, and that we learn from our mistakes. Adults need to model this understanding by openly learning from *their* mistakes.

One of my young patients was having a hard time getting off steroids—which he was using for athletic performance. He came into my office one day and said, "I'm quitting for good." When I asked what changed, he told me his basketball coach recently told him about his own mistakes with drug use in sports. Because he was bonded to his coach and admired his athletic abilities, he was determined to learn from his coach's mistakes and not do the same.

It Has to Come from Within

The bottom line is that people simply want to direct their own lives. We want our autonomy, mastery, and purpose—and these can't be imposed on us from the outside by anyone, not even parents. They're as individual and unique to ourselves as our fingerprints.

Self-motivation is necessary for our children's health, happiness, and success. Self-motivation is fueled by three things: (1) a balanced way of life that leads to autonomy, mastery, and purpose, (2) the ability to adapt to real life's ups and downs through CQ (which is why we need to live in the real world), and (3) a sense of internal control which comes from balanced authoritative parenting. Can you see how the imbalance of tiger parenting backfires when it comes to self-motivation and independence?

Through role modeling, guiding, and balanced living, dolphin parents demonstrate self-motivation in ways tiger parents can't. By being collaborative versus authoritative, supportive versus imposing, guiding versus directing, and responsive versus insensitive to our children's stage of change, we can empower our children and draw out their personal potential.

All that said, every single one of these behaviors won't produce a compliant child. Compliance is for tigers. Engagement is for dolphins. With engagement may come ambivalence and resistance, which are perfectly normal responses from children. After all, how many children *want* to study, practice piano, help with the dishes, *and* clean up their room? But the parenting journey will be so much more satisfying if you can ride these waves knowing that the outcome—fully developed self-motivation—will make your children's (and your own) lives so much happier and more successful.

Guiding Towards Twenty-First-Century Success

We know that supporting children's autonomy and limiting our interference results in better academic and emotional outcomes,[20] and that's exactly what dolphin parents aim to do. Now that you have established a balanced life, moved shoulder to shoulder with your children, and understand self-motivation, you are swimming towards the four Cs of CQ, adaptability, independence, and twenty-first-century success. The prescriptions that follow can help you along the way.

PRESCRIPTION

Make Learning Fun!

Fun can be a powerful teaching tool. One way to enhance the learning experience is to bring positive emotions into the task. We all know intuitively that working with someone who is in a good mood is much more motivating than working with someone who is in a bad mood. So how about just looking at a cute picture before a task? Japanese researchers tested a group of students on a dexterity task before and after showing them pictures of cute babies, puppies, or kittens. They found that the positive emotion triggered by the "cuteness" of the brief image was enough to improve performance![21]

Many children dislike math drills, and growing up we were no different. My dad knew this and used play and fun to teach math to his five children, whose ages spanned across twelve years. Dad could do a pretty good headstand, but to our delight, he would exaggerate his effort with facial contortions and near-tipping-over antics, which we all found hilarious. This was his secret fun weapon, and he used it to teach math. Often, after a long shift driving his taxi, dad would come home tired, but with pockets full of change. He would do his headstand in the living room, and we would all drop everything and gather around him. We would call out prime numbers and square root equations, and he would just jiggle his legs to release a few coins for each right answer. The total would be split among us. We knew he would tire within minutes, so we had no time for debate or squabble, only creative collaboration (my older siblings held up their fingers to help me out). Now, decades later, I still love math and will always remember that 157 is a prime number—with a huge smile on my face.

PRESCRIPTION

Provide Selective Positive Reinforcement for Positive Behaviors

All animals, including humans, benefit from positive reinforcement—especially when the reinforcing comes from someone with whom there is a personal connection. Exciting research on the use of positive reinforcement for childhood stuttering has turned the whole treatment field upside down. Historically, a speech therapist would break down words and parts of speech the child who stutters is having trouble with. The speech therapist would spend hours retraining the child to say these words and phrases correctly. Now, new methods point to simply using positive reinforcement for correct phrases and *completely ignoring* incorrect patterns of speech. The results are dramatic, especially when parents are trained to implement this technique on a daily basis. A direct *negative* correlation exists between how fast children's stuttering improves and how much they're corrected—meaning that the more focus is placed on the mistakes, the more mistakes children will make![22] But this treatment method is very different from praising just for the sake of praising, which has definite drawbacks, as the next prescription indicates.

PRESCRIPTION

Avoid Excessive or Empty Praise and Emphasize the Process, Not the Outcome

Carol Dweck, a psychology professor at Stanford University, found that people fall into two basic psychological mindsets: fixed and growth.[23] The fixed mindset is encouraged by excessive praise or emphasizing correct answers only. These children come to believe that they're "smart" or "talented," and are thus less likely to take risks that may shatter that fixed belief. They may be less curious and ask fewer questions because not knowing something doesn't fit their paradigm. They may also be less willing to tackle more difficult challenges, as these invariably involve making mistakes.

In contrast, Dweck found that those with growth mindsets are more willing to "stretch themselves to learn new things. They take on challenges, they stick to them, and they bounce back from failures."[24] The growth mindset is encouraged by empathizing effort, problem solving, consistency, and process.

In an experiment that demonstrates fixed versus growth mindsets and the downsides of "empty" praise, young children were asked to solve a simple puzzle, which most did with little difficulty.[25] But then Dweck told a few, but not all, of the children how very bright and capable they were. As it turns out, the children who weren't told they were smart were more motivated to tackle increasingly difficult puzzles. These children showed greater progress and interest in puzzle-solving, and also displayed higher levels of confidence. They enjoyed the thrill of choosing to work simply for its own sake, regardless of the outcome.

Although it may seem counterintuitive, providing non-specific praise for children's abilities and outcomes seems to rattle their confidence. However, if you stress *how* a child arrived at an answer and not whether the answer is correct, she will be more likely to make the effort, take risks, and try new ways of doing things. For example, if you appreciate the *effort* your child put into solving a math problem, as opposed to applauding the answer, she'll be more likely to learn from the experience and try it again.

My older son got into the habit of counting his soccer goals and announcing them to the world (likely because of our excessive praise and mindless encouragement of outcome, not process). However, it became clear that his focus on goals began to affect his performance in defense, passing, and setting up plays. The focus on goals was actually hurting him as a developing player. Although it's hard to resist applauding a goal, we now try our best to focus more on effort in the game. This small change helped our son be more present in the entire game and round out as a player. Based on the dolphin KEYS, we said, "Of course it feels great to score a goal [empathize], but you want to become a better player and support your teammates [identify your child's goals]. If you pay attention to more than just goals, you will definitely do both [support success]."

PRESCRIPTION

Let Your Child Try First Before You Step in and Provide Feedback

Watch your child try something *before* giving any instruction or advice. Afterwards, point out what he did correctly and what he needs to do to succeed. Then, have him try again. Repeat this process until he can solve the problem on his own. If the task is complex or time sensitive, ask him to describe how he would solve it first. Whenever I asked my supervisor at Harvard how to do something, he always made me do it first—even if I had no clue where to start. It would frustrate me to no end, as I had traveled across the continent for his instruction, not to muddle through things myself! However, once I ran into problems with something I tried on my own first and came back to him, he took the time to help me understand where my logic was flawed and asked me to try it again from that point. Through this process, I learned complicated research techniques very fast and also saw his efforts to bring out my own skills, which added to my desire to work harder and figure out things on my own.

My son used to always want help with his homework before he even tried it. I explained that homework isn't about getting the answer right or wrong—it's about figuring out what you need to learn and what you already know. Using my dolphin KEYS, I told him, "I know it's easier if I tell you how to do this [empathize], but that's not going to help your independence [identify your child's goals]. I'm sure you'll figure it out if you spend a few more minutes trying on your own [support success]." I also told him that "the whole point of homework is to just practice, make mistakes, and figure out what you need to learn." I had to say all this for almost every day for two weeks, but like a good politician, I stuck to my script and kept repeating myself, no matter what antics he tried to use to get me to help him first. Eventually, he realized that I was never going to help him until he tried his homework first. Guess what? When his younger brother came to him for help on his homework, my older son delivered my script perfectly!

PRESCRIPTION

Help Break Down a Problem Instead of Solving It

Suppose, for example, that your child is frustrated over a particular homework problem that she's been trying to solve. Instead of showing her how to do the whole thing, ask her where she's stuck and why. Then, encourage her to *break down* the homework problem into small steps. If you must, give a clue or small suggestion. As she progresses through resolving the problem, say things like "you're really close" or "I can help you with this, if you try that" (if she gets stuck).

Chloe loved science, but she was socially anxious. The science fair was coming up and her teacher suggested that she submit her project, but Chloe flat out refused. Her dad wanted to encourage Chloe to register, but he didn't want to push or hover. Using his dolphin KEYS, he said, "I can see you're feeling shy about registering for the science fair [empathize], but you also told me you don't want being shy to hold you back [identify your child's goals]. You love science so much, this is something you can do [support success]! I really think you should sign up for the science fair, but I certainly can't force you to do it." Once Chloe realized she was in control, she was open to telling her dad all the obstacles she expected to encounter with her project. He didn't solve each one for her, but he guided her on how to solve them herself. For example, she said she was nervous about talking about her project in front of strangers (that is, the judges), so he suggested other ways she could present her project, such as in print, as art, or in a video presentation. Chloe liked the idea of a video presentation but didn't know how to do it. Her dad then broke down that process for her and guided her on how to record her presentation on video. He also let her borrow his laptop to play it at her station. Chloe's father became a guide and teammate—not her director—for the project. The project was still hers, and so was the joy she received in presenting it.

PRESCRIPTION

Allow and Encourage Reasonable Risks

Hockey great Wayne Gretzky was fond of saying, "You miss every shot you don't take." The same is true for learning opportunities: if you don't try something, you'll never know what you may be missing out on. For example, your hockey-playing son may think he would not like yoga, but once he tries it, he may find that it's a great addition to his fitness schedule. Guide him to be curious, try new things, and take some risks.

Anika is twelve years old, is cautious, hates "new things," and is risk averse. As a result, she won't go to the park, her neighbor's homes, or school events. Her parents want to guide her towards exploration and taking some risks. Using their dolphin KEYS, they told her, "Yes, it can be really scary to take risks [empathize]. But there are so many things you want to do [identify your child's goals] that involve stepping out of your comfort zone. We know you can do it and are here to help you [support success]. Should we give it a try?"

Anika's dolphin parents got Anika's permission to gently nudge her out of her comfort zone. They asked her from which point on her street she would be comfortable walking home and then dropped her off a few houses away from that comfort zone every day after school. Each day, although she was a bit nervous, she found the walk home more and more manageable. Anika's parents were strong in their goal of increasing comfort with exploration, but they were also flexible when Anika was feeling overwhelmed or tired. After the first month, Anika loved the feeling of independence and trust from her parents. By the end of the year, Anika was walking the seven blocks home from school by herself. She confidently manages a street with major traffic, walks by strangers, and even runs some errands, such as picking up milk from the grocery store on the way home. Because of her newfound comfort with exploration, Anika has asked if she can join a school play and participate in social events that she had refused to engage in before.

PRESCRIPTION

Do Nothing—Let Your Child Experience Natural Consequences

If you employ the dolphin strategies on a daily basis, you'll be well on your way to helping your child develop strong self-motivation and CQ. But sometimes the waters get choppy, and you need a special tool to deal with problems that arise. Everyone has this special tool on hand: it's called *do nothing*. It's important to give children the opportunity to experience the natural consequences of their behavior rather than rescue them from such consequences.

A high level of distress may actually motivate a person towards positive action. The distress may be the consequence of being unmotivated. For example, failing an exam may lead a child to distress that "my teacher will think I'm not very smart," "my parents will take away my video games," or "I just feel terrible about not having tried hard enough." Any or all possible consequences may be enough to prompt the child to study more for the next exam (that is, the distress can lead to a change in behavior). The cognitive understanding of the benefits and drawbacks of a particular behavior—learned by the child through natural consequences—can turn a child towards or away from that behavior. The child who says, "I don't like doing homework, but I know the pros outweigh the cons" has gained a personal and meaningful grasp of how actions and their consequences can affect his own life and self-interests.

Yes, we can still take away video games, cancel a promised treat, or provide appropriate incentives. But we can't do these kinds of things forever, so it's best not to rely on them as primary or sole strategies. As hard as it may be for you to tolerate, if and when distressing events (such as getting caught cheating) occur, the natural consequences usually prove to be far more effective at helping a child develop an internal locus of control to avoid such events in the future.

The earlier in life you allow your child to experience natural consequences, the less devastating those consequences will be. In grade one, my oldest son didn't finish his first homework assignment, and I had the strong urge to rescue him. I was tempted to drop every-thing I was doing and sit down with him to get it done. Even though I wanted him to make a good first impression on his new teacher, I managed to stop myself. The next day, my son rushed home and started doing his homework right after school. Apparently, his teacher kept him in during recess to finish it, making him miss his beloved fifteen minutes of soccer time with his friends. I just got out of the way, and didn't yell or rescue, and he found his own motivation to get his homework done. Ah, the power of natural consequences!

So as you can see, the dolphin way honors our biology and serves our deepest human values. The dolphin way is intuitive, but not obvious if we're in fear mode. It's simple but not easy. And the simplest things in life are the most powerful—and totally worth it!

Chapter 10

WHAT HAPPENS TO CHILDREN
RAISED THE DOLPHIN WAY?

Isabella, a spunky and somewhat quirky seventeen-year-old, was referred to me because her parents were upset that she was skipping school, was getting lower grades, and was generally unfocused. Previously, Isabella had been an honor roll student.

When Isabella first came to me, she was on a math and science track at school and seemed irritable, glum, and withdrawn. I asked her what, if anything, she liked about school. She said she liked her one elective, drama class, "a bit." I asked her to tell me more, and she began to talk about how she liked the challenge of acting in different roles. As she spoke, she started to make eye contact with me, sat up straighter, and became more engaged. By the time she got around to telling me that she was good at acting and that it was the only thing she has ever really loved, she was fully lit up with excitement. But suddenly she started crying uncontrollably, saying that her parents would never accept her love of acting. "They want me to be a doctor or something." (I know. Sounds terrible, doesn't it?)

I assumed that pursuing the arts held some sort of stigma for Isabella's parents. You can imagine my surprise when I met her parents—*both* of whom are actors who had met onstage! In fact, the whole family was filled with actors and performers.

Despite their love of their profession, Isabella's parents thought she was "smart enough" to become a doctor; they hoped that she would end up in a more "secure" line of work than theirs, one where she wouldn't have to cope with the competition and sometimes random luck that typically rule an actor's life. All reasonable points, but what Isabella's parents hadn't considered was that their daughter had zero interest in math, science, or medicine. She was unhappy—and rebelling—because she was bored with her other classes and anxious because she was being turned away from her true passion.

Now, fourteen years later, Isabella is thriving. Her parents stopped pushing the sciences and gave her the green light for the arts. But even though Isabella took a lot of acting classes, she was influenced by her parents' guidance and didn't become an actor—at least not in the traditional sense. She found her very own path. Isabella picked a law class in first year university where she discovered the drama of the courtroom—and to her surprise and everyone else's, she went to law school.

Once she became a lawyer, Isabella explored and experimented with different theatrical styles in the courtroom to present arguments and win over juries. She developed so many of her own creative methods that, even at her young age, she is frequently invited to speak to other lawyers about courtroom performance. She has also found her way on television as a media expert on legal issues. Isabella has a vibrant and successful career as a lawyer. And she's healthy and happy to boot.

I'm sure Isabella could have made it through medical school—she did well in her science classes despite her obvious lack of interest. But what's better—an average and not so happy doctor or an extraordinary and happy lawyer? Isabella was able to connect with her *BEST self*.

Being your BEST self means having both a talent *and* a passion or spirit for something, as well as the self-motivation to act on your unique qualities (BEST = *B*est *E*xpression of one's *S*pirit and *T*alents). In my view, living your BEST self means applying the full potential of your mind, body, and spirit to its best possible use.

I often talk with my children—and anyone else who will listen—about the importance of living your BEST self. I recently had an exchange with my seven-year-old son that told me that he could see the use of the idea, even for books. One of the sofas in our house had a broken leg. My husband put some books underneath it to prop it up until it was fixed (which in our house, may be never). My son asked me why the books were there, and I explained to him that they were there to hold up the sofa. "But Mommy," he said, "that's not the best way to use the books. Why would you do that to those books?" He was right; the books would do an OK job as a substitute leg, but they weren't designed for that purpose, and it wasn't their best use.

So many people who come to my office are just like those books propping up my sofa. Their unique gifts and passions have been literally squashed by the weight of what they've been pushed to do. Clearly, the brain isn't just some lump of clay that can be molded in any way a parent chooses. It's the most complex thing in the known universe. Countless neuronal connections encode a functional map from which passions, talents, and motivation emerge.

The Building Blocks of a Healthy, Happy, Self-Motivated, and Fully Successful Life

It may come as no surprise that when you're your BEST self, you have the best chance of being healthy, happy, and self-motivated. I think we're fascinated by dolphins because their best selves are in line with what we envision our BEST selves to be. In the wild, tigers are also their best selves, but humans don't want to spend their lives like tigers—in solitude, sleeping most of the day so they can save energy for their big kill at night. We *want* to play, explore, hang out with our pod, give back to our communities and beyond, and have the same sense of joy that dolphins appear to have when they jump out of the water with their seemingly perpetual smiling faces.

As I've said all along, it's really difficult to be happy and self-motivated if you're not healthy—and your best chance for that comes from balancing the basics in life.

After health comes play. Play allows us to identify what we're passionate about, what our strengths and weaknesses are, and what we love and don't love. Having a spirit or passion for an activity makes you want to keep trying even when you're frustrated. After all, we're hardwired to want to challenge and excel—but not just at anything. We want to excel at those personal interests that are part of our spirit.

By playing and exploring in our youth, we can find our BEST self in adulthood. Being our BEST self in adulthood allows us to keep playing and exploring—including in our workplace. If Isabella's parents prevented her from exploring the world of theater, and if Isabella hadn't played by doing a lot of acting, she never would have discovered what made her tick. She would have been stuck in the world of science and medicine, which would not have afforded her the opportunity for happiness and true success.

After play and exploration come community and contribution. Because we're wired to be social, without community and contribution, our BEST self lies dormant without anyone to share it with. Playing with friends or sharing our lives with others adds to the joy and depth of our experiences. This is not to say that we can't find joy by doing things on our own. But if we choose to be overly competitive at the expense of being community-minded, we can't attract or keep close bonds. We may achieve social status, but we won't experience close and meaningful social bonds. As I showed in Chapter 7, being isolated or alone for any length of time is as damaging as severe illness.

Without the support of Isabella's acting community (and her contributions to that community), she may have never continued to pursue her passion, which led her to become her BEST self. Once her family came around to supporting her, she was able to feel the joy of sharing her life with them—a life they had particular love for and insight into. Without the support of her pod and without her vision of herself as part of a larger cast, Isabella would have never experienced happiness and success like she did.

After community and collaboration comes self-motivation. Here's what's so great: if we have balance and find our BEST selves or something close to it, drive is often completely—and effortlessly—internalized. We don't need anyone to push us because we're doing what we're curious about and what we want to do. We have all the motivation inside us that we need to push on and adapt, even when things get tough.

Isabella had to be pushed, prodded, and hovered over by her parents when she was doing science. The moment she switched over to what she loved doing, they didn't have to say a single thing to motivate her. They did have to make sure they stood shoulder to shoulder with her and didn't fully occupy the space of planning for her future so she could step into it herself.

The only way Isabella got to this place is through balance. First, balanced parenting allows for internal control. Second, a balanced way of life allows for health and internal drive. And what all of this leads to is a balanced brain, which is key to developing CQ. But before we get to further details on CQ, let me briefly explain how a balanced brain leads to health, happiness, motivation, and true success.

A Balanced Brain

Most of the body's paired organs—lungs, breasts, kidneys—perform identical functions, providing a backup should one side fail. Not so with the brain's two halves.

Our left brain is considered the logical, analytical brain. It is good at one-point focus, separateness, and "breaking things down." The left brain filters out information to find "usefulness" and is explicit. The process of language and logic occur in the left brain and it functions to provide sequences and plans. In general, the left brain has "positivity"—meaning it has a plan or direction.

In contrast, the right brain is considered our emotional, intuitive brain. It is good at holistic focus, "oneness," empathy, and "big picture" thinking. The right brain takes in information from the body and the environment to find "connection" and is implicit. The meaning of language such as the understanding of metaphor occurs in the right brain, and it functions to provide purpose and meaning.

So can you see how each of our hemispheres is not just different from but in fact a perfect complement for the other? If left brain is strength, right brain is flexibility. You could say that our knowledge accrued from academic learning (or "book smarts") is left brain and our knowledge that comes from real life experiences (or "street smarts") is right brain. So, of course, we are at a disadvantage if we operate from just one side of our brains. We need both left and right sides, *linking with* the positive aspects of the other and also *inhibiting* the other's reactive tendencies that most often come from fear.

Are the hemispheres in perfect balance? Or are they like the body, where even though we may be left- or right-side dominant, overall balance comes from integration, communication, and constant calibration among all parts? Controversy exists over left- or right-brain dominance. Until relatively recently, the left hemisphere was accepted as the dominant or major hemisphere, and the right brain was accepted as the subordinate or minor hemisphere. After all, the modern world clearly values logic and analysis over emotion and intuition—doesn't it? That's why we need scientific studies to "prove" that fresh air and sunlight are good for us! What's amazing is that on one hand (or from the left brain), you may logically agree with that statement. However, on the other hand (or from the right brain), you may also intuitively disagree with that statement. It seems that our left and right brains are constantly duking it out! But between the two, the right hemisphere may be running the show more than we once thought. Albert Einstein knew this and said, "The intuitive mind is a sacred gift and the rational mind is a faithful servant. We have created a society that honors the servant and has forgotten the gift."[1]

Since the left side of our body got our beautiful heart, perhaps it's only fair that the right side of our body gets the dominant emotional, intuitive brain. However, we now know that every type of function, including reason, emotion, language, and imagery, is served not by one hemisphere alone, but by an integration of both. Think about it this way: if our right brain is EQ, our left brain is IQ. However, the integration of both sides of the brain leads to what we truly need in this rapidly changing twenty-first century: CQ. Critical thinking requires seeing the big picture *and* the separate pieces. Communication requires logistics *and* the emotion of language. Collaboration requires the ability to be separate *and* connected. And creativity requires all hemispheric functions—explicit and implicit—to work together. When the hemispheric processes are integrated in this way, we excel in CQ and can constantly adapt. Please don't forget our all-important neuroplasticity: the ability for the brain to adapt in form and function. By living a life of balance and integration, our brains will develop balance and integration.

High CQ

To review, the four *C*s of CQ are creativity, critical thinking, communication, and collaboration. CQ doesn't just happen nor can it be imposed; it must be developed from within. If you're externally motivated, your chances of developing high CQ will plummet. The higher your CQ, the more adaptable you are. The more adaptable you are, the healthier, happier, and more successful you are. Remember that George Vaillant's Grant Study of Adult Development (in Chapter 3) identified mature adaptive style as a key determinant of success.

Let's look at how the components of CQ apply to our children's future success and happiness.

Creativity and Critical Thinking

"He outsmarted us," said Kelly Jakkola, the research director of the non-profit Dolphin Research Center in the Florida Keys. Jakkola was referring to Tanner, a bottlenose dolphin, who was asked to mimic his trainer's behaviors while he was blindfolded. Even though Tanner couldn't see his trainer's behaviors, he found a creative solution to the problem: he made sounds in the water and through echolocation, he identified his trainer's movement and then replicated them perfectly![2]

A lot of people believe that you're either born creative or you're not. In reality, creativity is less about what you're born with and more about what you *do* with what you're born with. The data are pretty clear on this point: many scientists have studied this question extensively and have concluded that about 70 percent of general intelligence (IQ) is purely genetic. However, creativity is only 30 percent genetic; the remaining 70 percent comes from your environment and *how* you learn.[3] In other words, it comes out of the *process* of learning. According to Robert Epstein, author of *The Big Book of Creativity Games*: "There's not really any evidence that one person is inherently more creative than another."[4] Instead, he says, creativity is something that anyone can cultivate, and that is exactly what happens through play and exploration.[5]

Another common assumption is that creativity is strictly related to the arts—music, theater, and literature. Sure, the arts are creative, but not every artist is creative. For example, some young musicians—maybe your own children—have incredible technical abilities but lack soul in their playing. In contrast, some math students who enjoy the subject area can create something truly inspiring from numbers and symbols.

Being creative can mean producing something new—a new symphony, a new novel, or a new way of doing math. But often it means simply engaging with something that already exists in a way that feels gloriously *different*. An actor doesn't have to rewrite Shakespeare's *Romeo and Juliet* to bring down the house, and a conductor doesn't have to revise Beethoven's Fifth Symphony to make the music feel new and fresh. Creativity can be about applying your passion to an existing activity to make an original contribution to the world.

Another common, yet false, assumption is that business is the antithesis of creativity. After all, could anything be *less* creative than supply, demand, profits, and financial reports (although every time a new financial scandal arises, we hear a lot about "creative accounting"!)? The business world is constantly adapting to changes in consumer demand and the economic world. Businesses create original new products often, but more often than not, a "new" product is a mix of features of existing products or an innovative twist on an existing product. Most people would agree that Steve Jobs was one of the most creative people of our time. But he didn't invent the personal computer, the cellphone, or the tablet computer. What he did, however, was apply his creativity to make each of these products better.

At some point, the line between critical thinking and creativity blurs, and solving problems becomes synonymous with thinking creatively. Critical thinking involves analyzing large amounts of information—including contradictory ideas and ideas that challenge our own ideas—and filtering out the bad from the good; finding patterns and drawing conclusions; and keeping an open mind and a healthy sense of skepticism. In our increasingly interconnected, 24/7 world, it's especially important to be able to interpret data from a wide variety of perspectives, some of which may be very different from our own. A truly critical thinker is comfortable with giving up past assumptions, embracing "what ifs," honestly exploring new ideas, and thinking outside of the box. Critical-thinking skills are nurtured by the freedom to question—not by passive instruction.

Creativity and critical thinking require a balanced state of mind. Lack of free time, stress, and external pressure are all well-known creativity killers. In contrast, sleep, play, and social partnership are powerful enhancers of creativity and critical thinking.

Sadness, fear, anger, and anxiety block creativity. A study of undergraduate students showed that sadness led them to fear mistakes and hold back new ideas.[6] Improved mood is clearly linked to enhanced creativity and critical thinking, such as generating answers to divergent thinking tasks, producing new endings to stories, making unique word associations, and even solving moral dilemmas.[7] Karen Gasper, a leading researcher on creativity, says that when you feel stuck or unmotivated, "take a walk, see a comedy, go out with a friend ... these breaks may help you feel better and see your work in a new light."[8] These findings sound like prescriptions for exercise, play, and community to me!

The relationship also runs in reverse. Creativity alone is linked to higher job satisfaction, higher quality leisure activities and experiences, increased feelings of positive emotions, greater overall well-being, and happiness. Research shows that people are more likely to have a creative breakthrough if they are happy the day before.[9]

Today, creativity may not only increase our happiness but also help us get a good job. In a recent survey published by the *Harvard Business Review*, 1,500 of the best-performing CEOs in the world identified creativity as the *number one leadership competency of the future*.[10]

Communication

Scientists have long debated whether dolphins' amazing collection of whistles, squeaks, barks, clicks, pops, and other sounds are complex enough to be an actual language. But there's no debate that dolphins use these sounds—along with body language—to communicate. Every dolphin has a unique "signature" whistle that identifies him or her to others. Dolphins also have a remarkable capacity for mimicking such sounds as motorboats and even human laughter. Dolphins' communication skills enable them to organize groups to hunt for food or to defend the pod from predators such as sharks. Communication is definitely going on while dolphin parents are showing their young how to protect themselves, hunt, and thrive in the wild.

Of all the CQ skills, communication is the most important for interacting in today's world. While all animals need to communicate effectively to survive, human beings, who are the most social of animals, need it the most. You may be super smart, an out-of-the-box thinker, and emotionally intelligent, but without the ability to express yourself in an effective and interesting way, no one will ever know your many talents.

Effective communication can vastly improve your leadership skills, as it gives you the ability to motivate and adequately convey your message to others. Good communication helps you avoid and handle stress, and increases your ability to connect with others, including friends and significant others.

In a society in which electronic communication is prevalent, those who can powerfully communicate both in person and online will stand out and be the leaders of tomorrow.

Communication begins with good listening skills—not just for content but even more so for emotion. So if you grew up never really being listened to, it's hard to know how to listen well. That's why it's so important to learn communication as a child. Many aspects of communication, especially non-verbal communication, are intuitive. Subtle behaviors—such as eye contact, nodding, smiling, a pat on the back, or the occasional affirmative statement—indicate that you're paying attention. However, they must come naturally or they become a distraction to communication. In fact, if we really don't believe what we're saying, our non-verbal signs will "tell on us" by sending unconscious contradictory messages. For example, saying that you're "really open to that idea" while your arms are crossed and as you lean back is a communication contradiction. However, you can consciously use your body language to strengthen your thinking—such as purposely standing tall, with shoulders back when you're nervous. In doing so, you will *look* more confident and also *feel* more confident as your brain and body are in constant communication themselves!

Communication skills develop over a lifetime of play, exploration, community, and contribution. Have a look at Table 10.1. It's a list of the applied skills employers consider "very important" for job success for new graduates who are entering the workforce. You'll notice that a few of these "very important" skills are communication related.

Table 10.1 Applied Skills Employers Consider "Very Important" for Job Success for New Graduates

Skill	Percentage of Employers Who Say It's Very Important
Oral communication	95%
Teamwork/collaboration	94%
Professionalism/work ethic	94%
Written communications	93%
Critical thinking/problem solving	92%
English language	88%
Ethics/responsibility	86%
Leadership	82%
Information technology	81%
Creativity/innovation	81%
Lifelong learning/self-direction	78%
Diversity	72%

Source: Conference Board of Canada, *Are They Really Ready to Work?* Ottawa: Author, 2006. Table 2, p. 20. http://www.p21.org/storage/documents/FINAL_REPORT_PDF09-29-06.pdf.

While some schools, colleges, and universities still emphasize test scores and grades, college graduates are being thrown into a work world that emphasizes CQ skills for which they may have had very little training.

Collaboration

Dolphins are famous for their collaborative way of life. While hunting with their pod, they often surround a school of fish and squeeze them into what's called a *bait ball*. Then, one by one, individual dolphins take turns plowing through the "ball," feeding on the stunned fish. Without this kind of collaboration, dolphins wouldn't be able to survive. We can't survive without collaboration either, even if we think we can—which is typically the case if we've grown up with tigers.

By working with others towards a common purpose, we can generate better ideas and find better solutions to problems. Whether with siblings, friends, classmates, or co-workers, we have numerous opportunities to collaborate. Collaboration is more than just working with others, however. It involves being respectful, reliable, and competent; using our social skills; and motivating, challenging, and inspiring one another. Collaboration skills are deepened by spending time with, working with, and exchanging ideas with diverse people in diverse situations. Collaboration is the foundation for social bonding, which definitely makes us happy!

One of the first places children can deeply explore collaboration is in the classroom. Many twenty-first-century classrooms around the world are moving towards greater collaboration. As long as the teacher remains a dolphin (and not a tiger or permissive jellyfish), these classrooms offer real advantages:

- *Shared knowledge among teachers and students.* In a collaborative classroom, the flow of information between teachers and students isn't unidirectional. Yes, teachers know more about a given subject, but students with some practical experience or ideas can contribute to the process of learning. What could be a better confidence builder than teaching something to your own peers?

- *Shared authority among teachers and students.* Shared authority allows students to take some responsibility for their learning. By participating in setting goals and time-lines and establishing milestones, some shared authority teaches children the very same skills they'll need to master in the independent workplace in the not-too-distant future.

- *Teachers who guide rather than direct.* When knowledge and authority are shared by the teacher and students, the teacher can become more of a guide than a director. Students are encouraged to solve problems independently and use creativity and critical-thinking skills to explore alternative solutions. Of course, the teacher is still available to gently nudge, redirect, explain, and even take control when needed.

If our children are going to be able to function in a collaborative world as adults, they have to learn how to collaborate when they're young. Since our children spend so much time in school, the classroom offers a great opportunity to teach and foster collaborative skills.

At school, children who act out on other children get in trouble. In the workplace, anyone who's ever had a co-worker who can't (or won't) get along with others knows that you're often left to figure out how to work with the miserable person on your own. It's no wonder that the ability to collaborate—especially with a diverse group of people—is a skill that's highly ranked by employers.[11]

Dolphins: Successful with a Capital S

Did you notice that Table 10.1 includes each skill that makes up CQ? Creativity, critical thinking, communication, and collaboration (plus other dolphin attributes such as ethics/responsibility and lifelong learning/self-direction).

In the work world, CQ skills are often referred to as "soft skills." The twenty-first-century workplace is increasingly complex, diverse, interdependent, and connected. People with "soft skills" typically have strong social skills; work well on diverse teams; communicate with clarity; quickly adjust to changes in human resources, technology, and workplace conditions; find creative solutions; and are able to innovate.

All of these soft skills add up to strong leadership—the elusive quality everyone is looking for. So who in the twenty-first century has strong leadership? Is it the overcompetitive tiger? The crispie? The teacup? No way! In the twenty-first century, it's the dolphin. The dolphin CQ skills of creativity, critical thinking, communication, and collaboration are definitely part of strong leadership. However, when these skills are combined with the dolphin character traits of empathy, community-mindedness, and altruism, the dolphin becomes unstoppable and successful with a capital *S*. Some of the traits linked to leadership are integrity (doing the right thing even if no one is watching), responsibility (being accountable to others and yourself), respect (showing it to even those who are different from you in views or opinions), empathy (trying to understand others from their perspective), and citizenship or altruism (working for the greater good).

Strong, successful lives thrive on all of these CQ-related characteristics: trustworthiness in the job, home, and community; respect for family, friends, colleagues, and neighbors; responsibility for the task at hand; and fairness towards others. In addition, exceptional lives happen when you exhibit the caring and sense of citizenship with others that dolphins exemplify. The phrase "nice guys finish first" is true and is the essence of competitive altruism. As a society, we value those who think of others first. Studies of altruism show that individuals who choose group over personal benefits gain reputation and status.[12]

Humans are social beings. And because of technology, the world has become smaller. Thus, in many ways, our future will be even more social. This fact provides dolphins with a competitive edge. The dolphin way is sustainable and a win-win: dolphins make great contributions to their communities, but they also thrive by doing so.

You may be thinking, *I know a lot of so-called successful people that have no soft skills whatsoever—people who work eighty hours a week, never play, are not creative, and are only focused on themselves.* Yes, tigers find success as well, but only in its most limited definition. I see these "success" stories every day in my office. And their "success" is accompanied by imbalance that can lead to depression, heart disease, immoral behavior, addiction, and death.

The tiger's definition of success usually involves achievement limited to career and wealth, whereas the dolphin's definition includes health, happiness, integrity, social bonds, community connection, and contribution. I know that on a superficial level, society rewards the tiger's definition of success by giving career and wealth along with considerable esteem. We have all heard someone say, "Mr. X is really successful," but that statement doesn't mean Mr. X is happy, a good father, highly creative, or helps others. It often just means that he has a lot of money. In fact, Mr. X could even be an unprincipled jerk.

Remember that dolphins have much higher expectations for their children and know that those who achieve success in *all* aspects of their life do so by maintaining their balance. They sleep, exercise, play, explore, bond socially, contribute, and are self-motivated. We don't hear as much about these success stories because the lack of drama doesn't make for good news. In contrast, cocaine addicts and abusive bosses make for great dirt. That's why we constantly hear about these problems but rarely hear about those who live healthy and happy lives. Maybe that's changing. The *Huffington Post* recently launched the blog "The Third Metric—Redefining Success beyond Money and Power" to accompany a conference of the same name. The blog focuses on redefining success to include health, happiness, and giving back to our communities.[13]

Finding Happiness as a Dolphin

Happiness is perhaps what parents want most for their children. Strangely, for tiger parents, happiness seems to be an after-thought. Tiger parents focus their efforts on the tools they think their children will need to compete for the material prizes in our society; once they've achieved the security of a high-paying job, they're free to seek happiness wherever and however they like. Therein lies the problem. Tiger parents make the false assumption that happiness is *not* necessary to achieve success in adult life and that their children can somehow figure out how to "obtain" happiness once they're adults. We know that childhood lays the foundation for all aspects of adult life. We know that an unhappy childhood is a risk factor for numerous psychological issues—difficulty with relationships, self-insight, and coping with stress, just to name a few.[14] An unhappy childhood also predisposes individuals to physical health issues such as heart disease, inflammatory conditions, and accelerated cell aging.

What is happiness? Many have pondered this question and there are diverse answers. Let's first look at what happiness is *not*.

To begin with, let me make a distinction between happiness and mental health. Mental health problems such as depression, anxiety, and substance use aren't synonymous with *unhappiness*, although they may be correlated with it. Depression is a medical condition that involves a constellation of symptoms such as impaired sleep, lack of concentration, failing memory, loss of energy, flagging interests, appetite dysregulation, and a low or irritable mood. Once the symptoms are treated, a person who has experienced depression may have a greater sense of happiness similar to someone who has recovered from a serious illness.

Happiness is unequivocally *not* money. Today, it's not always easy to distinguish between our needs and wants, and we often think that more or better things will mean more happiness. But, as we now know, this isn't the case. A recent report showed that once a person in the United States earns $75,000 per year, incremental increases in wealth don't affect happiness; some studies put the magic number at $50,000 per year.[15] In addition, although the United States has seen a steady rise in its GDP for the last three decades, there has been no correlating rise in the population's sense of happiness or well-being. More money, a bigger house, a fancier car, more gadgets, and designer clothes add no value to happiness. A famous study performed in 1978 measured the happiness levels of lottery winners against those of lottery non-winners and accident victims. Lottery winners were no happier than the control group of non-winners and accident victims; lottery winners actually found less pleasure in everyday events.[16]

When I was in my twenties, I took time off medical school and worked in an impoverished rural area of India right before I interned at the prestigious headquarters of the World Health Organization in Geneva. To me, the poor of India were clearly happier than the rich of Geneva. Despite the poverty, disease, and corruption in the rural Indian villages I worked in, the people's sense of joy and vitality was remarkable. Maybe that joy and vitality is driven by gratitude for what one has and optimism for the future. Consider the fact that citizens of African countries, many of which are among the world's poorest countries,[17] consistently rank among the most optimistic people in the world. A fifty-three-country Gallup poll rated Nigerians at seventy points for optimism. In contrast, Britain scored a deeply pessimistic negative forty-four.[18] These results show me just how powerful perspective can be. We all know that feeling stuck and constrained is frustrating, whereas having a positive view will bring us motivation and feelings of excitement. Citizens in difficult places to live (such as Nigeria) can accept that they have no control over their personal circumstances, but they can always control how they *perceive* those circumstances. We always have control over our point of view. When we look at the world knowing that we control our feelings and behavior, we benefit with less stress, improved life satisfaction, and even a longer life.[19] Perhaps the trouble lies in our difficulty in distinguishing between needs and wants. If so, happiness becomes a victim of economic well-being for those who equate more "things" with a better life. Remember affluenza? It's especially toxic to children. Why? Overindulging children with material goods can often lead children towards wanting more material rewards and away from pursuing what will make them truly happy—a balanced life with a sense of purpose or well-being.

The relationship between status and happiness is complicated. The desire for status motivates us to "climb the social ladder" and to want the esteem of others. Striving for the esteem of others is a good thing in that it can support the development of our honesty, ethics, and caring. However, caring too much about status and fearing the loss of status can cause what I believe is a key driving force behind tiger parenting: status anxiety.

If happiness isn't a lack of depression, or having money or status, then what is it exactly? In July 2011, the United Nations General Assembly passed a resolution encouraging countries to promote the happiness of their citizens.[20] A follow-up conference, called Happiness and Well-being: Defining a New Economic Paradigm, was held at UN headquarters in New York in April 2012, involving world leaders and global experts from a wide range of fields. The goal was to initiate next steps towards realizing a new global perspective that would include such measures as Gross National Well-being and Gross National Happiness. Conference participants explored the factors influencing well-being and happiness and came up with criteria to be measured when assessing a nation's well-being and happiness. Much debate took place over how to define happiness. Of course health—both physical and mental—came first with specific mention of sleep, nutrition, and exercise. Themes of a balanced life were prominent, with the use of time being "one of the most significant factors in quality of life—especially time for recreation and socializing with family and friends."[21] After this came "community vitality," including affectionate community relationships and practices of giving and volunteering. Of course, play and participation in cultural events and opportunities to develop artistic skills were also considered to be important factors. These are all core features of dolphin parenting—the basics of balance—health, play, community, and contribution.

Figure 10.1 presents Abraham Maslow's famous hierarchy of needs theory (the pyramid you might recall from Psych 101), which also exhibits many of the same findings from the conference. If you look at the categories within each need, you'll notice a lot of overlap with the dolphin way.

Figure 10.1 Maslow's Hierarchy of Needs

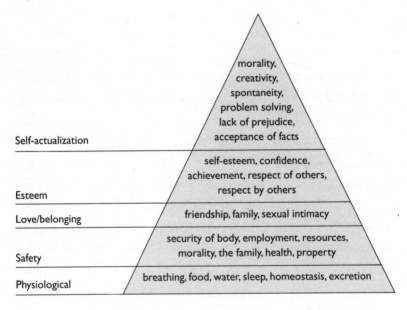

Maslow's simple but elegant five-stage model lays out the pattern of human motivations, from the motivation to satisfy the most basic needs of existence to the highest level of the hierarchy, where creativity, problem solving, spontaneity, and morality are essential needs for happiness.

The fulfillment of these needs is part of a balanced life. When we honor our basic survival and health, play freely, explore bravely, bond socially, contribute wholeheartedly, and challenge continuously, we create the foundation for the essential determinants of happiness.

Interestingly, a comprehensive study of well-being in Britain and the United States shows that happiness changes over a lifespan and follows a U-shaped curve.[22] Many of us parents are at an age at which we're at the bottom of the curve. Life satisfaction is at a minimum at ages forty-nine and forty-five for American males and females, respectively, with similar data (forty-four and forty-three, respectively) for European males and females. After the dip, it's possible that the upswing of the U-curve is explained by individuals relinquishing aspirations from their youth, which can lead them to enjoy life more.[23] I often wonder how being at your lowest point in life satisfaction while raising children affects their future happiness.

Perhaps, then, one of the best gauges for your child's chance for happiness is to ask yourself: *Am I happy?* So many of the unhappy teenagers I work with have parents who seem stressed and overwhelmed (in my opinion, often due to a tiger lifestyle). These teenagers say, "Do I really want to be like them?" and "If I do everything my parents want me to do, all this practicing, studying, etc., I will end up where they are and that is NOT where I want to be." For this reason, I urge all parents who want their children to be happy to make happiness a priority for themselves. The first step is moving towards a balanced way of life.

Putting It All Together

"Happiness is not something readymade. It comes from your own actions,"[24] said His Holiness Tenzin Gyatso, the fourteenth Dalai Lama.

Aaron was referred to me when he was thirteen. He was showing a progressive lack of interest in things, his grades were dropping, and his pediatrician wondered if Aaron could be depressed.

As usual, I began by taking a history. The further I went, the more I realized that Aaron wasn't actually clinically depressed but certainly unhealthy, unhappy, and not on track for success. When I asked about things he found stressful in his life, Aaron ticked off a list: "My science teacher sucks, my debate competition is coming up, everything is boring, and my parents are always interfering with my life."

I offered my usual reply. "Thanks. Got it. Anything else?"

After a significant pause, during which Aaron figured out I was willing to wait forever for his reply, he added softly, "Yeah. My brother, Adam, made it onto the varsity rugby team."

"OK," I said, "now rank each item of stress on a scale of one to ten, with ten being the most stressful."

Here's how Aaron ranked each item. Science teacher = nine: "My teacher is totally ruining the one subject that I liked. She just pushes facts down our throats, does no experiments, and hardly allows any questions." Debate competition = four: "I'm not that stressed about it. If I practice a bit more, I'll be fine. I'm good at debating, but it doesn't make me happy." Everything is boring = nine: "Now that science is ruined, I find nothing really interesting. It's so pointless anyway. All this work just to end up like my parents—unhappy and running around like they're on a hamster wheel." Brother making the varsity rugby team = ten: no comment.

Later, in a separate session, I asked Aaron's parents to list what they thought was stressful for him and to rank each item. I call this the "matching game"; it often reveals misperceptions parents have about what might be distressing their child. Aaron's parents initially only identified his science teacher and the debate competition as potential stressors, so Aaron filled them in on his list so they could rank his additions as well. Here's how Aaron's parents ranked his stresses. Science teacher = five: "He's getting a good grade, so it can't be that bad." Debate competition = nine: "He must be stressed about it." Everything is boring (and his parents are no fun) = five: "He has everything he could want; we even just got him a new iPad!" Brother making the varsity rugby team = four: "He may be a bit envious."

When we cross-referenced the rankings, Aaron wasn't surprised by his parents' responses, but they were shocked by his—especially by the ten for his brother's making the varsity rugby team. They had automatically thought Aaron was jealous of Adam; they had even tried to comfort him by suggesting he should be proud of his brother because "you will make it onto the rugby team one day too." But jealousy was not the problem. The problem for Aaron was that he was worried about his older brother. He knew that Adam had secretly tried a cycle of steroids last year, and he was worried that now, with fifteen hours of rugby plus weight-training in addition to his already jam-packed academic load, Adam would unravel under the pressure. Already, Adam was showing signs of being stressed and more irritable. Most of all, however, and in addition to the worry, Aaron missed his brother deeply. Only two years apart, the brothers had slept in the same room and often the same bed since they were toddlers. They had played together as children and were essentially each other's best friend. Aaron wasn't jealous; he was sad and worried about his most meaningful human connection, and it was making him unhappy.

In response, Aaron moved towards rebalancing his life, and it made him feel better. Aaron's parents stopped hovering and directing so much in areas that Aaron showed and wanted independence in. However, at his request, they did help him communicate to his teacher his desire for a more creative experience in science class. With her collaboration, they found him an after-school science enrichment program led by graduate students from the local university. Aaron learned from them and also began designing simple experiments for grade one and two students. He made rockets out of Menthos candy and coke cans as well as paper airplanes; these activities connected him with the thrill of learning and the joy of sharing it with others. Aaron continued on the debate team but decided to wind it down a year later to allow more time for science.

Aaron's parents helped him and his brother find time together while they themselves took time to enjoy their hobbies: golf for dad and hiking in nature for mom. The whole family slowed down a bit and spent more time together. The brothers played basketball together once a week, and the family tried to eat dinner together a few times a week, but that was a challenge. What worked best was getting together on weekends and scheduling in Saturday-morning breakfasts. Even though everyone was exhausted by Friday, Aaron would sleep in his brother's room, and by morning they would both be complaining that the other was "hogging all the pillows." They wouldn't talk much, but Aaron said that just being near his brother helped untie that terrible knot in his stomach.

With time to play and explore, Aaron was finding his BEST self. With the experiments he was designing and sharing with others, and the rekindled bond with his parents and brother, Aaron was feeling happy. He was excited about doing something he loved and found that he became more engaged in all his school subjects as a result. His marks improved, and so too did his overall health and performance. In every way, Aaron (and his whole family) was happier.

As I've tried to show throughout this book, the way to foster success in our children's lives is not by giving them "the best of everything," but by equipping them with the qualities they need to become healthy, happy, self-motivated, and truly successful.

When I began this book, I sat down with parents and asked them to tell me, from the heart, what future they wanted for their children. Most parents talked about a combination of strong moral character, intelligence, creativity, contribution, love, success, and happiness. Those qualities sound much more like those of dolphins rather than tigers.

Chapter 11

GETTING BACK TO BEING HUMAN

My neighbor Kate came to visit me when my daughter was four weeks old. She brought me a delicious fruit salad, and I brewed my special chai tea. She picked up the baby, remarking on how calming it was to hold a newborn, while I enjoyed the adult company post-delivery.

As I boiled water for my tea and stretched my back, Kate expressed her exasperation over her sixteen-year-old daughter, Samantha. Kate was at the end of her rope, and Samantha was spiraling out of control. Despite being a talented gymnast and a straight-A student, Samantha was, in Kate's words, "losing motivation," unhappy, and lashing out at her parents.

The latest issue was that Samantha wanted to spend more time with her friends, including some "tree-hugging guy" she met while on a nature retreat. Kate felt that the time spent away from academics and practice was really hurting Samantha. Perhaps, most of all, Kate was panicked that with university applications coming up, Samantha would ruin all the hard work she had put in so far, and not make it into one of her top choices for schools.

In at least five different ways and at least five different times, Kate said, "I just don't know what to do!" I knew she wanted me to tell her what to do, as many parents do at such moments—especially because I'm an "expert" on teen motivation. But Samantha wasn't my child, I wasn't Kate, and their home wasn't mine. So, how could I possibly know what would work best for her and her family?

I try my best to practice what I preach. I try not to tell people what to do, but rather guide them to find their own motivations and solutions. I definitely had some ideas as to what might help and what might not help, but I also knew Kate could come up with her own answers. So I asked Kate, "Well, what is your intuition telling you?"

"I'm so confused," she lamented. "I thought I finally had some clarity, but then I read some mommy blog written by someone with a similar problem and that threw me off. So I don't trust what little intuition I have left."

All the while, Kate was doing something so beautifully intuitive that I almost had to laugh. She was gently rocking my newborn daughter in her arms. She was talking in a quiet, hushed voice, and each time my baby squirmed, Kate gently pressed her cheek against my baby's cheek. Every so often, she would sniff my baby's head and say, "Ah, that scent is so relaxing."

With my baby, Kate was following her own natural intuition so completely that she didn't even notice! When I pointed this out, she stopped, looked at my newborn, looked at me with a puzzled expression, and said, "Well, where has this intuition gone when it comes to my daughter?"

Of course, Kate's intuition hadn't "gone" anywhere. It was where it had always been and where it is for every parent: deep inside. I said this to Kate, who replied, "Right now, the only intuition I have is to lock Samantha in the house or send her to live with her grandparents in small-town Nebraska. That can't be right, can it?" No, it wasn't right. The intuition to lock Samantha in the house or send her away was a classic fight or flight response, driven by fear. The trouble is, when we're out of balance due to fear, illness, or loneliness, our intuition follows suit.

Intuition is knowledge without conscious processing, thought, or observation. In contrast, *instincts* are impulses to act without conscious processing, thought, or observation. Intuition and instincts are related and often used interchangeably. When I ask my patients about their *intuition*, I'm really asking them about both of these things: I want to unearth the innate knowledge that's causing them to act in a particular way.

The trouble with our instincts is that when we're out of balance, they tend to lead us in the wrong direction. Fear is one of the worst causes of instincts gone awry precisely because our brains are programmed to fight, freeze, or flee when we're scared. Fighting, freezing, or fleeing makes sense when you're faced with a life-or-death situation, but not when you're faced with teenagers doing what teenagers are meant to do (even though it may feel like a life-or-death situation!). What Kate needed was to connect with her intuition, which is never based in fear. Intuition is the innate knowledge gifted to us by nature that can only be accessed in a place of calm awareness. Instincts can be wrong, but intuition is always right.

I looked at Kate again, who, as she took a break from sounding off, rocked from foot to foot as my baby started to doze off. She was like a scale with two equal weights, slowly balancing itself out. Her shoulders, which had been virtually up to her ears, had dropped, and her brow, which had been deeply furrowed, relaxed.

I got out the fruit salad Kate had brought, poured two cups of chai tea, put out a bowl of nuts, and brought us each a glass of water.

"Before you do anything else, I want you to take a really deep breath," I said to Kate. She did, and her rocking motion evened out even more. "Now have something to eat and drink."

Kate admitted that she hadn't been sleeping well and was so stressed out all morning that she hadn't had a single thing to eat or drink. She sat down on the couch with my daughter deftly in one arm, her head gently leaning on Kate's shoulder (this was a woman who knew just what she was doing!). Kate drank a glass of water, savored the mix of fruits, and then nibbled on nuts.

"I really needed that," Kate said. "I didn't realize how hungry I was. I can't believe how much better I feel."

"Tell me about the idea you had before you read the mommy blog," I prompted.

Kate paused, looked anxious again, like she was debating whether to tell me what seemed like a really dumb idea. But now that she was more herself, she finally let it out.

"Well, I was sitting at my desk looking at the mountain of college applications, and I was thinking that Samantha would really have to kill herself (and the rest of us) to get into her top choices. And even then, it's a lottery whether she'd get in or not. The fact is, she needs to cut down the competitive gymnastics due to her tendonitis the doctor has been hounding us about— and we haven't done a thing because we know it will definitely diminish her chances of getting in somewhere good. But that's not the point. My realization—and I know how stupid this sounds—is that it doesn't really matter what school she goes to. They're all good! And I know she'll do great anywhere." Kate started to cry. And I felt the tears welling up inside me as well.

"I can't believe I just said that," Kate said once she got her breath back. "Not the part about her not getting in. But that I said I know she'll do great anywhere. I can't believe I've never said this to her. No one has! No wonder she's so uptight. The poor child is like Atlas with the weight of all our expectations on her."

Of course, Kate's intuition had kicked right in once she gave herself the opportunity to get back into balance. I didn't need to say a single thing to her about what to do. She figured it out all on her own. We humans are amazing!

Reconnecting with Our Intuition

The metaphors of the tiger and the dolphin don't represent a contrast between two different types of people per se. We're all dolphins when we're balanced and tigers when we're not.

Shaking off the tiger and bringing out the dolphin is a process, and just like any process, our motivation will vary. One day, I'll meet another dolphin mom and feel awesome about the choices I'm making. The next day, I'll meet a hard-core tiger mom who bares her teeth at me, and I'm frightened her children will eat mine, so I relapse. Then, the day after, I'll go teach at the university and validate for myself (yet again) that no one likes tigers (not even tigers like themselves), so I reset to dolphin mode. Fluctuating, stumbling, and downright falling is all part of the process. Paradoxically, the sophistication of our brains makes us particularly prone to shifting back and forth between balance and imbalance. Life would be so much easier if we were mice or reptiles! Even though the reptilian brain is pretty small in comparison with ours, reptiles will rarely abandon their young, but humans will. One possible explanation for this is that reptiles don't get mixed messages from their simple brains, whereas our highly complex brains confuse us all the time! Reptile brains work only on instinct, whereas our brains are far more sophisticated and when not integrated, mixed messages or individual parts can take over. For example, fear-induced instincts such as fight, freeze, or flight, driven by an area of the brain known as the amygdala, may cause us to ignore or devalue logical or emotional information coming from our prefrontal cortex (the thinking part of the brain). We may be so scared of a spider that we panic even though our logic tells us it's harmless. In contrast, what we learn in our environment (for example, at school, in society, and at home) can cause us to act counter to our most basic instincts to sleep, rest, and play.

Humans appear to be the only animals that don't sleep enough, don't drink enough water, don't eat a balanced diet, and do stupid and crazy things like texting while driving or *screaming* at our children to "CALM DOWN!!!!!!!" I just heard the story of a man who died while trying to break his own world record for speed on a motorcycle. Although he was virtually guaranteed of dying during his attempt to break his own world record, he felt compelled to go for it anyway. Only a human would do such a nonsensical thing.

Unlike lower life forms, we're meant to employ our intuition *with* knowledge that comes from higher-order learning in an integrated way. Intuition is based on knowledge that's innate *and* learned. Intuitive knowledge is fine-tuned over time through real-life experiences. Intuition is what tells a senior police officer that something doesn't add up at a crime scene. It tells an experienced cardiologist that a patient has heart disease without her taking a single test. It tells a teacher with twenty years of experience that a student has a different way of learning on the very first day of school.

Intuition requires the integration of the left and right hemispheres of the brain: the left side's focus and separateness must connect with the right side's empathy and oneness. Intuition also requires integration between the lower brain (amygdala) and the higher brain (prefrontal cortex). But intuition includes a whole lot more than just the brain. In fact, "the human intuition system" is believed to come not from one specific place in the brain but from the integration of our whole brain, and other body parts, including our heart and gut. It makes sense that the heart and gut are involved. After all, we actually experience a "gut instinct" or "know" something in our hearts.

Are you ready for some mind-blowing science? Growing evidence shows that the gut and heart actually have mini-brains of their own! The gut brain (or the enteric nervous system) consists of over one hundred million neurons in a mesh-like connection imbedded in the lining of the intestines. This "second brain," as it has been called, communicates with the central nervous system (the brain and spinal cord), but can also operate autonomously as it remarkably contains all the necessary types of neurons capable of integration. Over thirty different neurotransmitters are part of this system, most of which are identical to the ones found in the brain, such as dopamine and serotonin. In fact, 95 percent of the body's serotonin—a well-known modulator of sleep, energy, concentration, appetite, emotions, and mood—lies within the gut.[1]

In 1991, scientists showed that the heart has a complex system of neurons, neurotransmitters, proteins, and support cells that work like a brain and connect to or act independently of the cranial brain.[2] The "heart brain" has 40,000 sensory neurons involved in relaying information to the cranial brain, and the heart sends more information to the brain than the brain does to the heart. The heart brain has both short- and long-term memory, and the signals it sends to the brain can affect our emotional experiences. Perhaps the electromagnetic fields emitted by our hearts are the basis for how we intuitively know whether someone's energy is good or bad.

So how is everything connected? Neurons in the gut and heart communicate to the brain via a powerful pathway called the *vagus nerve*. The term *vagus* comes from the Latin root "to wander," such as a vagabond. This nerve pathway wanders around our body collecting and conveying sensory information about the state of our body's organs (such as the gut and heart) to our brain. In fact, about 90 percent of the fibers in the vagus nerve transmit information one way, from the gut to the brain.[3] Thus, the feelings that come from our gut and our heart may be more accurate than our cognitive interpretations of them. Our gut and our heart just know certain things first. For example, the vagus nerve runs though the throat and inner ear, and it can "hear" the fear in another person's voice before our brain does, even if that person looks perfectly calm. Studies that have examined blood flow in the brain through fMRI (functional magnetic resonance imaging) conclude that our peripheral (body) blood pressure rises *before* our brain blood pressure when we anticipate danger.[4]

Anxiety can cause a racing heart and stomach upset, and stress affects blood pressure and appetite. We thought these processes were unidirectional, from the brain to the body, not the other way around. We're at a new frontier of science that points to the endless possibilities about how exactly our body and mind connect and integrate to form our most trusted source of health, happiness, and success—intuition.

Even though our interpretation of intuition can certainly be wrong, our intuition is never wrong. It comes from a complex system of interconnected processes. Players include the logical, learning left brain; the emotional, intuitive right brain; the vagus nerve; the heart; the gut; our sensory environments; and other mirror neurons and their electromagnetic fields!

For most of our history, humans relied solely on intuition—integrating innate knowledge with what we learned from our immediate environment. Instead of surfing the Net for know-how, our hunter-gatherer ancestors learned about hundreds of plant and animal species, and which foods were edible, poison-ous, and medicinal. Anthropologists have described hunter-gatherer existence as the "only stable way of life humans have ever known."[5]

Our current era could quite possibly be the most unstable existence humans have ever known because we're often deeply out of touch with our intuition.

When our decisions are based on fear, we're in real trouble. Unfortunately, the challenges of the twenty-first century coupled with age-old parenting concerns incite fears, but perhaps those fears are far greater than what they need to be. As a result, our fears take hold of us, allowing our lower brain to essentially take the driver's seat and relegate many of our other drives—sleep, play, connection—to the backseat. What we may not realize is that by living in fear, we dysregulate ourselves so much that we then fail to recognize true danger. Take my patients with drug problems. Many of them are so far down the road of addiction that their very lives are at risk before their parents even notice. We also fail to recognize what we need as human beings: the basics for survival, play and exploration, and community and contribution. It's truly startling what distracted, overgathering, overprotective, and overcompetitive parents don't see even when it's right in front of them. Of course, parents are under extreme pressure, and under such circumstances, it's sometimes hard to take a deep breath, stay calm, and use intuition to focus on the "big picture" of what really matters. However, now more than ever, it's essential for us to do so.

Every day, as parents, we're faced with countless decisions.

Should I wake him up or let him sleep five more minutes? How should I handle the attitude my daughter is giving me as I rush her off to school? Should I ignore it this time? Should I tell her nicely that I'm doing her a favor by reminding her of her text-books or is today the day to set limits for a bad attitude? Should I stay at the office an hour longer to complete my work? Should I buy bread that's gluten-free, wheat-free, whole grain, seven grain, brown, white, or enriched? And on and on it goes. As parents, how can we logically think through all of the decisions we face on a daily basis? Well, we can't and shouldn't have to if we're connected to our intuition. The confusion that comes from feeling overwhelmed makes our lower brain kick into fear mode, enacting our instinct to fight, freeze, or flee. We can do much better and function with our whole brains within an awareness of our choices. When we smell a baby's head, kneel down and talk to our children, or spontaneously hug our children, we're connected to a level of innate intelligence we don't understand and don't really need to understand, any more than dolphins do. We can choose to cultivate our intuition and nurture our own true internal nature. Don't worry—you can still panic occa-sionally, which serves our lower brain, or read parenting blogs and books (thank you for buying this one!), which feeds our left brain. However, good decisions will come more easily and natu-rally if you balance and integrate all parts of the brain and body to focus on intuition.

Dolphins Parents: A Balanced and Holistic Approach

Dolphin parents strive to be balanced and holistic—they inte-grate their innate wisdom *with* the knowledge they acquire from their environment to follow their intuition. Dolphin parents know that twenty-first-century parenting can easily fall into a state of imbalance and, thus, so can our children. They may say to themselves, *Yes, I can see what everyone else is doing, but it just doesn't feel right to me, or make sense for my family.* Dolphin parents constantly adapt to an ever-changing world while honoring their biology and not compromising their values.

Let's review how dolphin parents navigate twenty-first-century parenting pressures.

- *Dolphin parents are authoritative rather than authoritarian.* Dolphin parents aren't intimidated by the generation gap that exists between themselves and their children and don't become permissive jellyfish or authoritarian tigers.
- *Dolphin parents embrace globalization.* Dolphin parents encourage their children to socialize, network, communicate, collaborate, compete, and connect with children of different cultures and from different countries. They know that the future will be evermore interconnected culturally and globally and that adapting to diversity in their neighborhood, school, and workplace will help build cultural intelligence.
- *Dolphin parents know that technology is here to stay.* Dolphin parents communicate with their children about the power and perils of technology and guide them towards using it appropriately and effectively. They encourage the use of technology in a balanced way and welcome its use to enhance CQ. They discourage technology use that's mindless, irresponsible, and imbalanced. Dolphin parents establish a healthy mindset for technology by setting limits and staying firm, yet still adapting to its rapid pace of change.

- *Dolphin parents use media for information and entertainment, with limits.* Dolphin parents realize that the twenty-four-hour news cycle, reality television, social media, and commercials all add fear and anxiety to our already stressful lives. They don't buy the latest parenting gimmick or sign up for the latest activity without taking a few deep breaths and considering the pros and cons, as well as their own values. If they're really confused or tempted by all the advertising and hype, they may ask a more experienced podmate for advice.

- *Dolphin parents who are single parents or have little family support make pod formation with others a priority.* Dolphin parents reach out to other pod members and collaborate around parenting activities, such as babysitting and driving to activities. They work creatively towards establishing a community and don't give up on this goal, even if it takes time. They're also in tune with their intuition and establish a sense of trust before they allow their children to be influenced by others.

- *Dolphin parents find ways to problem solve major work-life balance issues.* Dolphin parents don't allow themselves to burn out from both ends. They're OK with not being perfect, make steps to reduce their load, and ask for and give help when needed.

- *When it comes to school admissions, Dolphin parents hope and plan for the best.* For dolphin parents, the "best" school isn't necessarily the one with the highest ranking, but the school that's best for their child. That's the school that will best nurture their child's nature. They consider schools whose admission process *won't* destroy their child's health, happiness, self-motivation, or CQ. Dolphin parents know that childhood is the only foundation for life, so a balanced childhood with enough survival activities can't be compromised for anything—not even Harvard. Does this mean Dolphin parents shouldn't strive for top-tier schools? Absolutely not! Dolphin children "get in" all the time. They're the ones who know that the best way to excel in the short and long term is to maintain good health and balance, and use CQ to adapt.

Just for a moment, imagine where we would be as parents, where our children would be as independent adults, and where our world would be if the university admission process were different. Imagine what our collective future would be like if, after a certain academic standard, the *only* question for admissions was: "How have you made the world a better place?" Imagine all the time, money, energy, and resources being dedicated not towards a "fat envelope," but towards creating a better world. Would we not then see the true potential of the human mind and spirit? Would we not see a better world for all to live in?

- *Dolphin parents choose the dolphin way.* Dolphin parents use their intuition and, based on that, see their children for who they really are. They pay attention to the bond with their children and use it to effectively guide them. They maintain a balanced lifestyle themselves. They take deep breaths. They act on what they know: that balance, intuition, role modeling, and guiding are the most effective parenting tools. These tools are part of our biology and are what we're meant to do, driven to do, and rewarded for. The reward is the feeling of joy parents get when their children are healthy, happy, self-motivated, and truly successful. When "things don't feel right," they see it as a signal that they're going against their intuition and heading towards imbalance. Dolphin parents raise their children in the real world and constantly adapt to the changing real-world environment. They have the highest expectations for their children to succeed in all realms of life. They live a life and support their children in living a life that encompasses their full potential. Yet, despite these lofty goals, dolphin parenting is far simpler than tiger parenting. As you know, simple doesn't mean easy, but in this case it means the most powerful.

Throw Away Your To-Do List

What happens when we're balanced? We don't overschedule, overpush, overdirect, or overhover. We don't view life as a competition, but as a journey through ever-changing waters. We don't feel the pressure to keep up with the Joneses. We don't overgather, overprotect, and overcompete. We make sleep, a healthy diet, drinking water, being active, and deep breathing a priority. We understand that the world is changing and that it's necessary to adapt rather than to revert to a style of being that no longer fits our world. We value CQ over rote learning so that we can adapt and more fully inhabit what makes us unique and special. We value play and exploration just as much as we value traditional learning. We stay connected with and contribute to our community; by thinking beyond ourselves, we show our children how to relate to others, find their identity, build trust, gain respect, be responsible, and care about others and the world they live in. We let our children make their own choices—even if they might not be the best choices—because the locus of control and drive resides within our children, not within us. We allow not only our children but also ourselves to be healthy, happy, self-motivated, and successful.

Believe me, I know that all of this is much easier said than done. I sincerely hope this book hasn't left you feeling like you now have more things to add to your to-do list. Instead, I hope that I've helped you consider what's most important— those things that sustain us and come naturally if we just tune in. They don't need to be written down, and they don't require instructions.

This book can serve as a guide that you can come back to for support when you need it. With that in mind, let me leave you with a few last thoughts that may help launch you on your transformational journey of change.

First, any journey that requires change has bumps along the way. But with each bump that you weather, you become stronger and get closer to true transformation. With my patients, I talk about the following four stages of the journey, each of which gets you closer to transformation: *response, remission, recovery,* and *renewal.* For example, you may respond to this book by dimin- ishing your tiger behaviors right away. Then you may experience a remission, meaning the absence of tiger symptoms (but there is still risk of relapse). Then you may experience recovery; the tiger is gone for good and you find balance, who you really are inside, or your "old self again." If you really stick with a life of balance over the long term, you will find renewal, a sense of being better than ever, of true human vitality.

To help you get through these stages, do two things. First, find some podmates. Studies show that people generally benefit from going through a process of change with someone else (whether it's losing weight or quitting smoking). You may find some mates at www.thedolphinway.net, and I'll be there swimming along with you! Next, find a role model—someone you look up to as a parent and person. The role model could be a friend, an acquaintance, or a famous figure. A role model is someone you think of or call when you're stuck, or the person you think of when you ask yourself: *What would _____ do in this situation?*

Lastly, and most important, remember your true intentions as a parent: to raise a healthy, happy, and truly successful child. Health comes first because it's the basis for everything else in life. A balanced way of life is the best way to ensure good health. In our pressured world, both balance and health must be a clear goal for all parents and can't be taken for granted. Happiness comes next. It's simple: if your child is unhappy, so are you—and the ache doesn't stop until and unless you know your child is feeling well again. From the very first moment we become parents, our happiness is forever intertwined with that of our children. As you know by now, when I refer to success, I'm not talking about a single narrow definition of the term that will only get you a job in New York, London, or Hong Kong. Success is the culmination of health (physical, mental, and social), self-motivation, and happiness—that cherry on top that comes as a result of knowing who you are, who your community is, and how you can uniquely contribute to the world.

Whenever I get out of balance or get confused about my intentions in a situation, I think about my parents and their approach to parenting and life. I used to think my mom was a good parent despite the fact that she was so simple, had no education, and couldn't read. However, now I think she was a good parent precisely because she was so simple, had no education, and couldn't read. Perhaps this allowed her to maintain and develop the intuition she was born with—the knowledge and intelligence gifted by nature to all of humankind. In the face of her immensely stressful life, she was able to cut though all the noise and focus on what mattered the most because she used her intuition. She valued common sense and "street smarts" as much or more than book smarts. She never did anything that didn't "feel right" to her—especially when it came to how she raised her children. She grew up learning to look inward for the answers rather than outward, which gave her balance. My mom is a deeply spiritual person, and she calls her intuition her spirit. Whatever it is, or whatever you want to call it, the answer is always inside of us, even when the answer is that you need outside help or guidance. Whether you believe in a higher being, evolution, the universe, Mother Nature, or random chaos, we can all agree that all animals have a natural aptitude for knowing what to do.

Now that we know what we know, we don't really need the tiger or dolphin metaphor at all, because we humans are perfectly capable of being great parents—maybe even better parents than any other species due to our incredible and complex biology. We are naturally motivated. Moreover, health, happiness, and adaptability represent the human default position. Children have much to learn from their parents, but as parents, we have much to learn from our children. Children prove that vitality, love, and curiosity are natural in human beings. They also prove that we are all meant to sleep, move our bodies, play outside, explore our worlds, connect socially, and help one another. Our children remind us about the sheer joy of being. To be good parents, all we need to do is complement what we know with our intuition. With nature as our ally, we can lovingly guide our children towards health, happiness, and true success in all aspects of life. I don't think any other animal can make this claim.

NOTES

. . . .

Introduction

1. C. H. Kinsley and R. A. Franssen, "The Pregnant Brain as a Revving Race Car," *Scientific American*, January 19, 2010, http://www.scientific american.com/article.cfm?id=pregnant-brain-as-racecar.

2. "NAMI on Campus," The National Alliance on Mental Illness, accessed January 15, 2014, http://www.nami.org/Template .cfm?Section=NAMI_on_Campus.

3. "Mental Health: A Call for Action by World Health Ministers," World Health Organization, 2001, http://www.who.int/mental_health/ advocacy/en/Call_for_Action_MoH_Intro.pdf.

4. "'Get the Facts' Prescription Drug Abuse on College Campuses," National Counsel on Patient Information and Education, accessed January 15, 2014, http://www.talkaboutrx.org/documents/GetTheFacts.pdf; "State Estimates of Nonmedical Use of Prescription Pain Relievers," *The NSDUH Report*, January 8, 2013, http://www.samhsa.gov/data/2k12/ NSDUH115/sr115-nonmedical-use-pain-relievers.htm.

5. World Health Organization, "Suicide Huge but Preventable Public Health Problem, Says WHO," news release, September 8, 2004, http:// www.who.int/mediacentre/news/releases/2004/pr61/en/.

6. M. Quigley, "Educational Baggage: The Case for Homework," *REACT* 22 (June 2003), http://repository.nie.edu.sg/jspui/bitstream/10497/4088/ 1/2003Issue1.pdf#page=7.

7. http://quotationsbook.com/quote/32470/.

Chapter 1

1. K. Perry, "Ohio Judge Orders Stalking Parents Away from Daughter," *USA Today*, December 26, 2012, http://www.usatoday.com/story/news/nation/2012/12/26/judge-orders-stalking-parents-away/1791795/.

2. A. M. White and S. Swartzwelder, *What Are They Thinking?!: The Straight Facts about the Risk-Taking, Social-Networking, Still-Developing Teen Brain.* New York: W.W. Norton, 2013.

3. A. Hasham, "Survey: Teens on Facebook More Likely to Do Drugs." *Thestar.com.* August 25, 2011, http://www.thestar.com/life/parent/2011/08/25/survey_teens_on_facebook_more_likely_to_do_drugs.html.

4. K. Kross, P. Verduyn, E. Demiralp, J. Park, D. S. Lee, N. Lin, S. Holly, J. Jonides, and O. Ybarra, "Facebook Use Predicts Declines in Subjective Well-Being in Young Adults," *PLoS ONE* 8, no. 8 (2013). doi:10.1371/journal.pone.0069841.

5. American Academy of Pediatrics, "Children, Adolescents, and Advertising," *Pediatrics* 118, no. 6 (December 2006): 2563–2569. doi:10.1542/peds.2006-2698.

6. D. A. Christakis, "The Effects of Infant Media Usage: What Do We Know and What Should We Learn?" *Acta Paediatrica* 98, no. 1 (2009): 8–16. doi:10.1111/j.1651-2227.2008.01027.x.

7. U.S. Census Bureau, "Single-Parent Households: 1980 to 2009," U.S. Census Bureau, Statistical Abstract of the United States, 2012, http://www.census.gov/compendia/statab/2012/tables/12s1337.pdf.

8. "Half of Americans Bring Work Home." LiveScience.com, January 13, 2010, http://www.livescience.com/9796-americans-bring-work-home.html.

9. United Nations Population Fund, *State of the World Population 2007: Unleashing the Potential of Urban Growth.* New York: United Nations Population Fund, 2007.

10. E. B. Smith, "American Dream Fades for Generation Y Professionals," *Bloomberg News*, December 21, 2012, http://www.bloomberg.com/news/2012-12-21/american-dream-fades-for-generation-y-professionals.html.

11. C. Cakebread, "Boomerang Kids: 51 Percent of Canadians 21–24 Live at Home," *Chatelaine*, November 11, 2011, http://www.chatelaine.com/living/budgeting/boomerang-kids-51-percent-of-canadians-21-24-live-at-home/.

12. L. Lim, "And You Thought the Tiger Mother Was Tough," NPR, December 14, 2011, http://www.npr.org/2011/12/14/143659027/and-you-thought-the-tiger-mother-was-tough.

13. National Institute on Alcohol Abuse and Alcoholism, *Parenting to Prevent Childhood Alcohol Use*. n.p.: National Institute on Alcohol Abuse and Alcoholism, July 2013, http://pubs.niaaa.nih.gov/publications/adolescentflyer/adolFlyer.pdf.

14. "Overindulgent Parents Harm Their Children." Relationship Matters.com, July 11, 2010, http://www.relationshipmatters.com/overindulgent-parents-harm-their-children/.

15. J. Rigby, "Stop Overindulging Your Children," Family Life.com, accessed January 15, 2014, http://www.familylife.com/articles/topics/parenting/foundations/character-development/stop-overindulging-your-children.

16. A. Inoue and N. Kawakami, "The Japan Work Stress and Health Cohort Study Group, Interpersonal Conflict and Depression among Japanese Workers with High or Low Socioeconomic Status: Findings from the Japan Work Stress and Health Cohort Study," *Social Science & Medicine* 71, no. 1 (July 2010): 173-180, http://dx.doi.org/10.1016/j.socscimed.2010.02.047.

17. J. de Graaf, D. Wann, and T. Naylor, *Affluenza: How Overconsumption Is Killing Us*. San Francisco, CA: Berrett Koehler, 2014, 1.

18. A. De Botton, *Status Anxiety*. New York: Pantheon, 2004.

Chapter 2

1. W. Pei-Chang, T. Chia-Ling, W. Hsiang-Lin, Y. Yi-Hsin, K. Hsi-Kung, "Outdoor Activity during Class Recess Reduces Myopia Onset and Progression in School Children," *Ophthalmology* 120, no. 5 (May 1, 2013): 1080–1085. doi:10.1016/j.ophtha.2012.11.009.

2. "Physical Activity and Sedentary Behavior's Association with Body Weight in Korean Adolescents," Pubmed.gov, February 23, 2013, http://www.ncbi.nlm.nih.gov/pubmed/22805715.

3. "Students 'Drugged' in Class Ahead of Gaokao," *China Daily*, August 5, 2012, http://www.chinadaily.com.cn/china/2012-05/07/content_15227568.htm.

4. E. Yard and R. Comstock, "Compliance with Return to Play Guidelines Following Concussion in U.S. High School Athletes, 2005–2008," *InformaHealthcare* 23, no. 11 (2009): 888–898.

5. L. Bakhos, G. Lockhart, and R. Myers, "Emergency Department Visits for Concussion in Young Child Athletes," *Pediatrics* 126, no. 3 (2010):

550–556; http://www.cdc.gov/traumaticbraininjury/pdf/BlueBook_ factsheet-a.pdf.

6. "Academic Cheating Fact Sheet," Stanford University, accessed January 15, 2014, http://www.stanford.edu/class/engr110/cheating. html.

7. K. Lunau, "Campus Crisis: The Broken Generation," *Maclean's,* September 5, 2012, http://www2.macleans.ca/2012/09/05the-broken-generation/.

8. J. M. Twenge, B. Gentile, C. N. DeWall, D. Ma, K. Lacefield, and D. R. Schurtz, "Birth Cohort Increases in Psychopathology among Young Americans, 1938–2007: A Cross-Temporal Meta-Analysis of the MMPI," *Clinical Psychology Review* 30, no. 2 (2010): 145–154. doi:10.1016/j.cpr.2009.10.005.

9. Ibid.

10. J. Whitlock, J. Muehlenkamp, A. Purington, J. Eckenrode, P. Barreira, G. B. Abrams, T. Marchell, V. Kress, K. Girard, C. Chin, and K. Knox, "Nonsuicidal Self-Injury in a College Population: General Trends and Sex Differences," *Journal of American College Health* 59, no. 8 (2011): 691–698; K. Lunau, "Campus Crisis: The Broken Generation," *Maclean's,* September 5, 2012, http://www2.macleans.ca/2012/09/05/the-broken-generation/.

11. R. Grenoble, "Chinese Students Sign 'Suicide Waivers' Before Starting College," *Huffington Post,* September 18, 2013, http://www.huffingtonpost.com/2013/09/18/chinese-students-suicide-waiver_n_3948310.html.

12. X. Li, "On Chinese College Students' Suicide: Characteristics, Prevention and Crisis Intervention," *International Journal of Higher Education* 1, no. 2 (2012): 103, http://www.sciedu.ca/journal/index.php/ijhe/article/view/1579/810.

13. M. McDonald, "Elite South Korean University Rattled by Suicides," *New York Times,* May 22, 2011, http://www.nytimes.com/2011/05/23/world/asia/23southkorea.html?pagewanted=all&_r=0.

14. A. Mukherji, "Student Suicides Soar 26% in 5 Years, Education System Blamed," *Times of India,* November 2, 2011, http://articles.timesofindia.indiatimes.com/2011-11-02/india/30349474_1_student-suicides-education-system-higher-education.

15. S. Y. Kim, Y. Wang, D. Orozco-Lapray, Y. Shen, M. Murtuza, "Does 'Tiger Parenting' Exist? Parenting Profiles of Chinese Americans and

Adolescent Developmental Outcomes," *Asian American Journal of Psychology* 4, no. 1 (2013): 7–18.

16. Ibid.

17. USC Center for Enrollment Research, Policy, and Practice, *A Call for Individual and Collective Leadership.* Los Angeles, CA: USC Center for Enrollment Research, Policy, and Practice, 2011, http://www.usc.edu/programs/cerpp/docs/CERPP_ConferenceReport_FINALforprint.pdf.

18. Ibid.

19. Ibid.

20. IBM, *Capitalizing on Complexity.* Somers, NY: IBM, 2010, http://public.dhe.ibm.com/common/ssi/ecm/en/gbe03297usen/GBE03297USEN.pdf.

21. J. Twenge, E. C. Freeman, and W. K. Campbell, "Generational Differences in Young Adults' Life Goals, Concern for Others, and Civic Orientation, 1966–2009," *Personality Processes and Individual Differences* 22, no. 5 (2012): 1045–1062, http://www.apa.org/pubs/journals/releases/psp-102-5-1045.pdf; A. G. Walton, "Millennial Generation's Non-Negotiables: Money, Fame and Image," *Forbes*, March 19, 2012, http://www.forbes.com/sites/alicegwalton/2012/03/19/millennial-generations-non-negotiables-money-fame-and-image/.

22. "The 'Millennials' Are Coming," *60 Minutes*, May 23, 2008, http://www.cbsnews.com/news/the-millennials-are-coming/.

23. Jason Dorsey, interview on *The Early Show*, CBS, November 13, 2011, http://www.youtube.com/watch?v=K7HiQxnLMyo&feature=related.

24. S. Hofferth and J. Sandberg, *Changes in American Children's Time, 1981–1997.* Ann Arbor, MI: Populations Studies Center at the Institute for Social Research, University of Michigan Institute, 1999, http://www.psc.isr.umich.edu/pubs/pdf/rr00-456.pdf.

Chapter 3

1. CIA, The World Factbook, accessed January 25, 2014, https://www.cia.gov/library/publications/the-world-factbook/fields/2034.html.

2. *"Industry Overview—Synovate Report," Hkexnews.hk*, accessed January 15, 2014, http://www.hkexnews.hk/reports/prelist/Documents/EMOEDU-20110616-10.pdf.

3. A. Ripley, "Teacher, Leave Those Kids Alone," *TIME.com.* September 25, 2011, http://content.time.com/time/magazine/article/0,9171,2094427,00.html.

4. C. Kim, "Korean Tiger Moms Scrimp for Tutors in Blow to Spending: Economy," *Bloomberg.com*, June 14, 2013, http://www.bloomberg.com/news/2013-06-14/korean-tiger-moms-scrimp-for-tutors-in-blow-to-consumer-spending.html.

5. S. E. Abrams, "The New Republic: The U.S. Could Learn from Finland," *NPR*, January 28, 2011, http://www.npr.org/2011/01/28/133301331/the-new-republic-the-u-s-could-learn-from-finland.

6. F. Zakaria, "GPS Special—Restoring the American Dream: Fixing Education," *CNN*, June 11, 2011.

7. A. Taylor, "26 Amazing Facts About Finland's Unorthodox Education System,"*Business Insider*, December 14, 2011.

8. A. Bryant, "On GPAs and Brainteasers: New Insights from Google on Recruiting and Hiring," LinkedIn, June 20, 2013.

9. Ibid.

10. D. Wisenberg, "How Young Entrepreneurs Turned a Tweet from Richard Branson into $1 Million," *Entrepreneur*, July 11, 2012, http://www.entrepreneur.com/article/223954.

11. G. Mason, "UBC Moves to Broaden Student Population," *Globe and Mail*, September 10, 2012, http://www.theglobeandmail.com/news/british-columbia/ubc-moves-to-broaden-student-population/article1360143/.

12. Ibid.

13. Veritas Prep, "What Looming MCAT Changes Will Mean for Aspiring Doctors," *U.S.News & World Report*, March 5, 2012. http://www.usnews.com/education/blogs/medical-school-admissions-doctor/2012/03/05/what-looming-mcat-changes-will-mean-for-aspiring-doctors.

14. "A Brief History of the SAT and How It Changes," *Peterson's*. N.p., January 23, 2013. http://www.petersons.com/college-search/sat-scores-changes-test.aspx.

15. F. Di Meglio, "Want an MBA From Yale? You're Going to Need Emotional Intelligence," *Bloomberg Businessweek*, May 15, 2013, http://www.businessweek.com/articles/2013-05-15/want-an-mba-from-yale-youre-going-to-need-emotional-intelligence.

16. Ibid.

17. Ibid.

18. P. Wiseman, "Firms Seek Grads Who Can Think Fast, Work in Teams," *AP*, June 24, 2013, http://bigstory.ap.org/article/firms-seek-grads-who-can-think-fast-work-teams.

19. Ibid.

20. Ibid.
21. G. E. Vaillant, *Triumphs of Experience: The Men of the Harvard Grant Study*. Cambridge, MA: Belknap of Harvard University Press, 2012.
22. Ibid.
23. Ibid, 52.
24. M. Bardo, "Divided Dolphin Societies Merge 'for First Time,'" *BBC Nature News*, July 30, 2012, http://www.bbc.co.uk/nature/18985101.

Chapter 4

1. L. J. Nelson, L. M. Padilla-Walker, K. J. Christensen, C. A. Evans, and J. S. Carroll, "Parenting in Emerging Adulthood: An Examination of Parenting Clusters and Correlates," *Journal of Youth and Adolescence* 40, no. 6 (June 2011): 730–743, http://link.springer.com/article/10.1007/s10964-010-9584-8#.
2. D. E. Bednar and T. D. Fisher, "Peer Referencing in Adolescent Decision Making as a Function of Perceived Parenting Style," *Adolescence* 38 (2003): 607–621.
3. "Vitality," Dictionary.com, accessed January 15, 2014, http://dictionary.reference.com/browse/vitality.

Chapter 5

1. S. Tucker, "Two-Thirds of Americans Don't Drink Enough," Boston College, January 7, 2011, http://www.bc.edu/offices/dining/nutrition/topics/drinkenough.html.
2. "Adult Obesity," Obesity Prevention Source—Harvard School of Public Health, January 5, 2014, http://www.hsph.harvard.edu/obesity-prevention-source/obesity-trends/obesity-rates-worldwide.
3. "Silent Killer, Global Public Health Crisis," World Health Organization, April 3, 2013, http://www.who.int/campaigns/world-health-day/2013/en/.
4. G. Kolata, "For the Overweight, Bad Advice by the Spoonful," *New York Times*, August 30, 2007, http://www.nytimes.com/ref/health/healthguide/esn-obesity-ess.html; Y. Wang and M. A. Beydoun, "The Obesity Epidemic in the United States–Gender, Age, Socioeconomic, Racial/Ethnic, and Geographic Characteristics: A Systematic Review and Meta-Regression Analysis," *Epidemiologic Reviews* 29, no. 1 (2007): 6–28, http://epirev.oxfordjournals.org/content/29/1/6.full.
5. "The Global Burden of Disease Study 2010," *Lancet*, December 13, 2012, http://www.thelancet.com/themed/global-burden-of-disease.

6. "Eating Disorder Statistics," The Alliance for Eating Disorders Awareness, accessed January 15, 2014, http://www.ndsu.edu/fileadmin/counseling/Eating_Disorder_Statistics.pdf.

7. Ibid.

8. C. M. Shisslak, M. Crago, and L. S. Estes, "The Spectrum of Eating Disturbances," *International Journal of Eating Disorders* 18, no. 3 (1995): 209–219.

9. "Diversity: Eating Disorders Don't Discriminate," National Eating Disorders Association, accessed January 15, 2014, http://www.nationaleatingdisorders.org/diversity.

10. S. H. Kennedy, R. W. Lam, S. V. Parikh, S. B. Patten, and A. V. Ravindran, "Canadian Network for Mood and Anxiety Treatments (CANMAT) Clinical Guidelines for the Management of Major Depressive Disorder in Adults," *Journal of Affective Disorders* 117, Suppl. 1 (2009): S26–S43, http://www.canmat.org/resources/CANMATDepressionGuidelines2009.pdf.

11. "Generation M2: Media in the Lives of 8 to 18 Year Olds," Kaiser Family Foundation, January 2010, http://kaiserfamilyfoundation.files.wordpress.com/2013/04/8010.pdf.

12. C. E. Landhuis, R. Pulton, D. Welch, and R. J. Hancox, "Does Childhood Television Viewing Lead to Attention Problems in Adolescence? Results from a Prospective Longitudinal Study," *Pediatrics* 120, no. 3 (2007): 532–537. doi:10.1542/peds.2007-0978.

13. M. E. Schmidt, T. A. Pempek, H. L. Kirkorian, A. Frankenfield Lund, and D. R. Anderson, "The Effects of Background Television on the Toy Play Behavior of Very Young Children," *Child Development* 79, no. 4 (July/August 2008): 1137–1151.

14. Entertainment Software Association, "Sixty-Eight Percent of U.S. Households Play Computer or Video Games," news release, June 2, 2009, http://www.theesa.com/newsroom/release_detail.asp?releaseID=65.

15. Nielsen Newswire, "U.S. Homes Add Even More Sets in 2010," news release, April 28, 2010, http://www.nielsen.com/us/en/newswire/2010/u-s-homes-add-even-more-tv-sets-in-2010.html.

16. Ibid.

17. R. Nauert, "Dreams Are Key to Memory," PsychCentral, April 26, 2010, http://psychcentral.com/news/2010/04/26/dreams-are-key-to-memory/13157.html.

18. A. Novotney, "The Science of Creativity," *gradPSYCH*, January 2009, http://www.apa.org/gradpsych/2009/01/creativity.aspx.

19. U. Wagner, S. Gais, H. Haider, R. Verleger, and J. Born, "Letters to Nature: Sleep Inspires Insight," *Nature* 427 (January 22, 2004): 352–355, http://www.nature.com/nature/journal/v427/n6972/abs/nature02223.html.

20. S. Sharma and M. Kavuru, "Sleep and Metabolism: An Overview," *International Journal of Endocrinology* (April 28, 2010), http://www.hindawi.com/journals/ije/2010/270832/.

21. C. Guilleminault and S. N. Brooks, "Excessive Daytime Sleepiness: A Challenge for the Practising Neurologist," *Brain* 124, no. 8 (2001): 1482–1491.

22. M. W. Chee and W. C. Choo, "Functional Imaging of Working Memory after 24 Hr of Total Sleep Deprivation," *The Journal of Neuroscience* 24, no. 19 (2004): 4560–4567.

23. Hypertension/High Blood Pressure Health Center, "Hypertension Overview," WebMD.com, http://www.webmd.com/hypertension-high-blood-pressure/default.htm.

24. A. R. Wolfson and M. A. Carskadon, "Sleep Schedules and Daytime Functioning in Adolescents," *Child Development* 69, no. 4 (1998): 875–887, http://www.ncbi.nlm.nih.gov/pubmed/9768476.

25. "How Much Sleep Do I Need?" Centers for Disease Control and Prevention, November 13, 2013, http://www.cdc.gov/sleep/about_sleep/how_much_sleep.htm.

Chapter 6

1. P. Gray, "All Work and No Play Make the Baining the 'Dullest Culture on Earth,'" *Psychology Today*, July 20, 2012. http://www.psychologytoday.com/blog/freedom-learn/201207/all-work-and-no-play-make-the-baining-the-dullest-culture-earth.

2. Ibid.

3. S. L. Brown and C. C. Vaughan, *Play: How It Shapes the Brain, Opens the Imagination, and Invigorates the Soul.* New York: Avery, 2009, 112.

4. Brown and Vaughan, *Play: How It Shapes the Brain.*

5. Ibid., 9.

6. http://www.goodreads.com/quotes/286612-play-is-the-highest-form-of-research.

7. http://www.brainyquote.com/quotes/quotes/c/carljung125773.html.

8. "Play Science—The Patterns of Play," The National Institute for Play, accessed January 14, 2014, http://www.nifplay.org/states_play.html.

9. L. Cosmides and J. Tooby, *Evolutionary Psychology: A Primer.* Santa Barbara, CA: Center for Evolutionary Psychology, University of California, 1997, http://www.cep.ucsb.edu/primer.html.

10. "Play Science—The Patterns of Play."

11. Ibid.

12. F. R. Wilson, *The Hand: How Its Use Shapes the Brain, Language, and Human Culture.* New York: Vintage, 1999.

13. S. B. Kaufman, "The Need for Pretend Play in Child Development," *Beautiful Minds* (blog), March 6, 2012, http://www.psychologytoday .com/blog/beautiful-minds/201203/the-need-pretend-play-in-child-development.

14. M. Root-Bernstein, "Imaginary Worldplay as an Indicator of Creative Giftedness," *Psychology Today,* December 2, 2008, http://www .psychologytoday.com/files/attachments/1035/imaginary-worldplay-indicator-creative-giftedness.pdf.

15. "Play Science—The Patterns of Play."

16. "Play Science—The Patterns of Play"; Stuart Brown, "Play Is More Than Just Fun," TED Talks, May 2008. http://www.ted.com/talks/stuart_ brown_says_play_is_more_than_fun_it_s_vital.html.

17. "Play Science—The Patterns of Play."

18. R. Ahern, R. Beach, S. Moats Leibke, I. Proud, A.-M. Spencer, and E. Strickland, "The Benefits of Play Go Well Beyond Physical Fitness," *Exchange Magazine,* September 2011, https://secure.ccie.com/ library/5020168.pdf.

19. "Play Science—The Patterns of Play."

20. P. LaFreniere, "Evolutionary Functions of Social Play: Life Histories, Sex Differences, and Emotion Regulation," *American Journal of Play* 3, no. 4 (2011): 464–488.

21. Brown, "Play Is More Than Just Fun."

22. Brown, "Play Is More Than Just Fun"; M. Monroe, "What's Your Play Personality?" Empowered to Connect, accessed January 15, 2014, http:// empoweredtoconnect.org/whats-your-play-personality/.

23. D. Elkind, "Can We Play?" Greater Good, March 1, 2008, http:// greatergood.berkeley.edu/article/item/can_we_play.

24. Ibid.

25. Ibid.

26. B. Azar, "Its More Than Fun and Games," *Monitor on Psychology* 33, no. 3 (March 2002): 50, http://www.apa.org/monitor/mar02/morefun .aspx.

27. Brown and Vaughan, *Play: How It Shapes the Brain*.

28. "Charles Joseph Whitman," *Murderpedia*, accessed January 15, 2014, http://murderpedia.org/male.W/w/whitman-charles.htm.

29. "Play Deprived Life—Devastating Result," The National Institute for Play, accessed December 10, 2013, http://www.nifplay.org/whitman.html.

30. N. Shute, "Play Author Stuart Brown: Why Playtime Matters to Kids' Health and Brains," US News.com, March 9, 2009.

31. Brown and Vaughan, *Play: How It Shapes the Brain*, 43.

32. Ibid., 43.

33. Ibid..

34. H. Cooper, J. C. Robinson, and E. A. Patall, "Does Homework Improve Academic Achievement? A Synthesis of Research, 1987–2003," *Review of Educational Research* 76, no. 1 (2006): 1.

35. Brown and Vaughan, *Play: How It Shapes the Brain*, 48.

36. R. Louv, *Last Child in the Woods*. New York: Algonquin Books of Chapel Hill, 2005.

37. R. M. Ryan, N. Weinstein, J. Bernstein, K. W. Brown, L. Mistretta, and M. Gagné, "Vitalizing Effects of Being Outdoors and in Nature," *Journal of Environmental Psychology* 30, no. 2 (June 2010): 159–168, http://dx.doi.org/10.1016/j.jenvp.2009.10.009.

38. Ibid.

39. A. Cramb, "Jogging in Forest Twice as Good as Trip to Gym for Mental Health," *Telegraph*, June 20, 2012, http://www.telegraph.co.uk/health/healthnews/9344129/Jogging-in-forest-twice-as-good-as-trip-to-gym-for-mental-health.html.

40. Ibid.

41. "Spending Time in Nature Makes People Feel More Alive, Study Shows," University of Rochester, June 3, 2010, http://www.rochester.edu/news/show.php?id=3639.

42. Ryan et al., "Vitalizing Effects of Being Outdoors and in Nature," 159.

43. "Spending Time in Nature."

44. http://www.leadershipnow.com/creativityquotes.html.

45. J. Dyer, H. Gergersen, and C. M. Christensen, "Five Discovery Skills that Distinguish Great Innovators," Working Knowledge, Harvard Business School, July 20, 2011, http://hbswk.hbs.edu/item/6760.html.

46. B. Watley, "Failure Is the Entrepreneur's Best Friend," *BizNOW*, accessed January 25, 2014.

47. G. Wolf, "Steve Jobs: The Next Insanely Great Thing," *Wired*, February 1996, http://www.wired.com/wired/archive/4.02/jobs_pr.html.

48. "'You've Got to Find What You Love,' Jobs Says," *Stanford Report*, June 14, 2005, http://news.stanford.edu/news/2005/june15/jobs-061505 .html.

49. Ibid.

Chapter 7

1. Associated Press, "Dolphin Appears to Rescue Stranded Whales," NBCNEWS.com, March 13, 2008, http://www.nbcnews.com/id/ 23588063/ns/world_news-world_environment/#.Uubf7SKEiWg.

2. M. Caney, "Dolphins Helping Humans," Dolphin Way, April 12, 2011, http://www.dolphin-way.com/dolphins-%E2%80%93-the-facts/ dolphins-helping-humans/

3. E. Young, "Dolphin Mums Need Help from Their Friends," *Australian Geographic*, November 2, 2010, http://www.australiangeographic.com.au/ news/2010/11/dolphin-mums-need-help-from-their-friends/.

4. "Community," *Dictionary.com*, accessed November 4, 2014, http:// dictionary.reference.com/browse/community.

5. Walton, "Millennial Generation's Non-Negotiables."

6. G. MacDonald and M. R. Leary, "Why Does Social Exclusion Hurt? The Relationship between Social and Physical Pain," Psychological Bulletin 131, no. 2 (2005): 202–223, http://www.sozialpsychologie.uni-frankfurt .de/wp-content/uploads/2010/09/MacDonald-Leary-20051.pdf.

7. D. Yates, "Researchers Look for Ingredients of Happiness around the World." *News Bureau Illinois*, June 29, 2011, http://news.illinois.edu/ news/11/0629happiness_eddiener.html.

8. Ibid.

9. E. W. Dunn, L. B. Aknin, and M. I. Norton, "Spending Money on Others Promotes Happiness," *Science* (March 2008): 1687–1688, https:// www.sciencemag.org/content/319/5870/1687.short.

10. D. Rico, "The Science of Giving: Why Giving Feels So Good," *Huffington Post*, January 11, 2012, http://www.huffingtonpost.com/2012/01/11/ the-gift-of-giving_n_1200238.html.

11. J. Moll, F. Krueger, R. Zahn, M. Pardini, R. de Oliveira-Souza, J. Grafman, "Human Fronto-Mesolimbic Networks Guide Decisions about Charitable Donation," *Proceedings of the National Academy of Sciences of the United States of America* 103, no. 42 (2006): 15623–15628.

12. J. Suttie and J. Marsh, "5 Ways Giving Is Good for You," UC Berkeley, December 13, 2010. http://greatergood.berkeley.edu/article/item/5_ways_giving_is_good_for_you.

13. Ibid.

14. "Cases of Collaboration and the Five Elements of Discovery," accessed January 15, 2014, http://128.143.168.25/classes/200R/Projects/Fall_1997/collaboration/tccprinciples.htm.

15. P. Deyell-Gingold, "Successful Transition to Kindergarten: The Role of Teachers & Parents," Earlychildhood NEWS, accessed January 14, 2014, http://www.earlychildhoodnews.com/earlychildhood/article_view. aspx?ArticleID=477.

16. S. Shalev, *A Sourcebook on Solitary Confinement*. London, UK: Mannheim Centre for Criminology, London School of Economics, http://www .solitaryconfinement.org/sourcebook.

17. J. Shulevitz, "The Lethality of Loneliness." *New Republic*, May 13, 2013, http://www.newrepublic.com/article/113176/science-loneliness-how-isolation-can-kill-you.

18. Ibid.

19. F. Fromm-Reichmann, *Loneliness*. Washington, WA: White Psychiatric Foundation, 1969.

20. Shulevitz, "The Lethality of Loneliness."

21. G. Anderson, "Loneliness among Older Adults: A National Survey of Adults 45+" AARP.org, September 2010, http://www.aarp.org/personal-growth/transitions/info-09-2010/loneliness_2010.html.

22. N. Eisenberger, J. M. Jarcho, M. Lieberman, and B. D. Naliboff, "An Experimental Study of Shared Sensitivity to Physical Pain and Social Rejection," *Pain* 126 (2006): 132–138; Shulevitz, "The Lethality of Loneliness."

23. R. McCraty, M. Atkinson, et al. "The Electricity of Touch: Detection and Measurement of Cardiac Energy Exchange Between People," (1996). Proceedings of the Fifth Appalachian Conference on Neurobehavioral Dynamics: Brain and Values, Radford VA, Lawrence Erlbaum Associates. Mahwah, NJ; R. McCraty, M. Atkinson, et al. "The Role of Physiological Coherence in the Detection and Measurement of Cardiac Energy Exchange Between People," (1999). Proceedings of the Tenth International Montreux Congress on Stress, Montreux, Switzerland.

24. Y. Sankar, "Character Not Charisma Is the Critical Measure of Leadership Excellence," *Journal of Leadership and Organizational Studies* 9, no. 4 (2003): 45–55, http://jlo.sagepub.com/content/9/4/45.short.

25. J. D. Creswell, W. T. Welch, S. E. Taylor, D. K. Sherman, T. L. Greunewald, and T. Mann, "Affirmation of Personal Values Buffers Neuroendocrine and Psychological Stress Responses," *Psychological Science* 16 (2005): 846–851.

26. http://gratituderadiostations.com/gratitude-research/.

27. J. Winifred, "Gratitude: Year-Round Attitude!" Psychcentral.com, November 21, 2012, http://blogs.psychcentral.com/wellness/2012/11/gratitude-year-round-attitude/.

28. R. A. Emmons, *Thanks! How the New Science of Gratitude Can Make You Happier*. New York: Houghton Mifflin, 2007.

Chapter 8

1. F. R. Niaraki and H. Rahimi. "The Impact of Authoritative, Permissive and Authoritarian Behavior of Parents on Self-Concept, Psychological Health and Life Quality," *European Online Journal of Natural and Social Sciences* (January 2, 2013), http://european-science.com/eojnss/article/view/24.

2. G. Dewar, "The Authoritative Parenting Style: Warmth, Rationality, and High Standards," Parenting Science, last modified March 2013, http://www.parentingscience.com/authoritative-parenting-style.html.

3. J. Gross, "What Motivates Us at Work? 7 Fascinating Studies That Give Insights," *TED* (blog), April 10, 2013, http://blog.ted.com/2013/04/10/what-motivates-us-at-work-7-fascinating-studies-that-give-insights/.

4. Dewar, "The Authoritative Parenting Style"; J. Krevans and J. C. Gibbs, *Society for Research in Child Development* 67, no. 6 (1996): 3263–3277, http://www.jstor.org/stable/1131778; A. Knafo and R. Plomin, "Parental Discipline and Affection and Children's Prosocial Behavior: Genetic and Environmental Links," *Journal of Personality and Social Psychology* 90 (2006), 147–164.

5. W. R. Miller and S. Rollnick. *Motivational Interviewing: Preparing People for Change*. New York, NY: Guilford, 2002.

6. W. R. Miller and S. Rollnick, *Motivational Interviewing: Helping People Change*. New York, NY: Guilford, 2013.

7. Ibid.

Chapter 9

1. "Professor Sir John Gurdon DPhil DSc FRS, Nobel Prize in Physiology or Medicine, 2012," *Gurdon Institute*, last modified October 9, 2012, http://www.gurdon.cam.ac.uk/jbg-report.html.

2. K. Cherry, "What Is the Difference between Extrinsic and Intrinsic Motivation?" *About.com*, accessed November 3, 2013, http://psychology.about.com/od/motivation/f/difference-between-extrinsic-and-intrinsic-motivation.htm.

3. "Stages of Change Model," University of Ottawa, Last modified July 31, 2009, http://www.med.uottawa.ca/sim/data/Stages_of_Change_e.htm; M. Gold, "Stages of Change," PsychCentral.com, accessed January 7, 2014, http://psychcentral.com/lib/stages-of-change; "The Stages of Change," Virginia Tech Continuing and Professional Education, accessed January 7, 2014, http://www.cpe.vt.edu/gttc/presentations/8eStagesofChange.pdf.

4. "The Stages of Change," Virginia Tech Continuing and Professional Education.

5. http://www.brainyquote.com/quotes/quotes/e/eleanorroo161633.html.

6. M. J. Kang, M. Hsu, I. M. Krajbich, G. Loewenstein, S. M. McClure, J. T. Wang, and C. Camerer, "The Wick in the Candle of Learning: Epistemic Curiosity Activates Reward Circuitry and Enhances Memory," *Psychological Science*, 20, no. 8 (2009): 963–973.

7. J. Lehrer, "The Itch of Curiosity," Wired Science Blogs/Frontal Cortex, August 3, 2010, http://www.wired.com/wiredscience/2010/08/the-itch-of-curiosity/.

8. http://www.wittyprofiles.com/q/3811156.

9. M. Popova, "Autonomy, Mastery, Purpose: The Science of What Motivates Us, Animated," Brain Pickings, accessed January 12, 2014, http://www.brainpickings.org/index.php/2013/05/09/daniel-pink-drive-rsa-motivation/.

10. Lehrer, "The Itch of Curiosity."

11. S. Dominus, "Is Giving the Secret to Getting Ahead?" *International New York Times*, March 27, 2013, http://www.nytimes.com/2013/03/31/magazine/is-giving-the-secret-to-getting-ahead.html?ref=magazine&_r=1&pagewanted=all&.

12. Ibid.

13. J. Lipman, "Why Tough Teachers Get Good Results," *Wall Street Journal*, September 27, 2013.

14. Ibid.

15. C. Bergland, "The Athlete's Way," *Psychology Today*, December 26, 2011, http://www.psychologytoday.com/blog/the-athletes-way/201112/the-neuroscience-perseverance.

16. Ibid.

17. A. L. Duckworth, "Angela Lee Duckworth: The Key to Success? Grit," TED.com, April 2013, http://www.ted.com/talks/angela_lee_duckworth_the_key_to_success_grit.html.

18. D. Pink, "Dan Pink: The Puzzle of Motivation," TED.com, July 2009, http://www.ted.com/talks/dan_pink_on_motivation.html.

19. Ibid.

20. M. Levine, "Raising Successful Children," *International New York Times*, August 4, 2012, http://www.nytimes.com/2012/08/05/opinion/sunday/raising-successful-children.html?pagewanted=all&_r=0.

21. J. Gross, "What Motivates Us at Work: 7 Fascinating Studies That Give Insights," TED Blog, April 10, 2013. http://blog.ted.com/2013/04/10/what-motivates-us-at-work-7-fascinating-studies-that-give-insights.

22. B. Guitar and T. J. Peters, *Stuttering: An Integrated Approach to Its Nature and Treatment*. Baltimore, MD: Williams & Wilkins, 1998.

23. C. S. Dweck, *Mindset: The New Psychology of Success*. New York: Random House, 2006: 248.

24. "Carol Dweck, Stanford University Professor, On Why Telling Your Children They're Smart Is Actually Bad for Them," *Huffington Post*, August 2, 2013, http://www.huffingtonpost.com/2013/08/02/carol-dweck-mindset_n_3696599.html.

25. Ibid.

Chapter 10

1. https://www.goodreads.com/quotes/7090-the-intuitive-mind-is-a-sacred-gift-and-the-rational.

2. S. Laboy, "Dolphins Problem-Solve Like Humans, New Study Shows (Video), *Huffington Post*, August 9, 2013, http://www.huffingtonpost.com/2013/08/09/study-dolphins-problem-solve-humans_n_3731435.html.

3. J. H. Dyer, H. B. Gregerson, and C. M. Christenen, "The Innovator's DNA," *Harvard Business Review*, December 2009, http://hbr.org/2009/12/the-innovators-dna.

4. R. Epstein, *The Big Book of Creativity Games*. New York: McGraw-Hill, 2000.

5. Ibid.

6. "The Science of Creativity." http://www.apa.org/gradpsych/2009/01/creativity.aspx.

7. K. Gasper, "Permission to Seek Freely? The Effect of Happy and Sad Moods on Generating Old and New Ideas," *Creativity Research Journal*, 16, no. 2 (2004), 215–229.

8. Novotney, "The Science of Creativity."

9. B. L. Fredrickson, *Positivity*. New York: Random House, 2009; B. Breen, "The 6 Myths of Creativity," *Fast Company*, December 2004, http://www.fastcompany.com/51559/6-myths-creativity.

10. "IBM 2010 Global CEO Study: Creativity Selected as Most Crucial Factor for Future Success." IBM, May 18, 2010, http://www-03.ibm.com/press/us/en/pressrelease/31670.wss.

11. Conference Board of Canada, *Are They Really Ready to Work?* Ottawa: Author, 2006. Table 2, p. 20. http://www.p21.org/storage/documents/final_report_pdf09-29-06.pdf.

12. C. L. Hardy and M. Van Vugt, "Nice Guys Finish First: The Competitive Altruism Hypothesis," *Personality and Social Psychology Bulletin* 32, no. 10 (2006): 1402–1413.

13. HuffPost's *The Third Metric: Redefining Success Beyond Money & Power*, http://www.huffingtonpost.com/news/third-metric.

14. K. Batcho, "Childhood Happiness: More Than Just Child's Play," *Psychology Today*, January 13, 2012, http://www.psychologytoday.com/blog/longing-nostalgia/201201childhood-happiness-more-just-childs-play.

15. D. Kahneman and A. Deaton, "High Income Improves Evaluation of Life But Not Emotional Well-Being," *Psychological and Cognitive Sciences*, July 4, 2010; J. Sanburn, "Why $50,000 May Be the (New) Happiness Tipping Point," *Time*, April 19, 2012.

16. P. Brickman, D. Coates, and R. Janoff-Bulman, "Lottery Winners and Accident Victims: Is Happiness Relative?" *Journal of Personality and Social Psychology* 36, no. 8 (1978): 917–927, http://www.ncbi.nlm.nih.gov/pubmed/690806.

17. "World's Poorest Countries," Infoplease, accessed January 14, 2014, http://www.infoplease.com/ipa/A0908763.html.

18. Ibid.

19. J. Rodin and J. E. Langer, "Long-Term Effects of a Control-Relevant Intervention with the Institutionalized Aged," *Journal of Personality and Social Psychology* 35, no. 12 (1997): 897–902.

20. United Nations, *World Happiness Report 2013*. New York: United Nations, 2013, http://unsdsn.org/files/2013/09/WorldHappinessReport 2013_online.pdf.

21. "Community Sustainable Happiness Week," The Happiness Initiative, 2011, http://www.happycounts.org/community-sustainable-happiness-week/.

22. D. G. Blanchflower and A. J. Oswald, "Well-being over Time in Britain and the USA," *Journal of Public Economics* 88 (2004): 1359–1386.

23. Blanchflower and Oswald, "Well-being over Time"; United Nations, *World Happiness Report 2013*.

24. http://www.brainyquote.com/quotes/quotes/d/dalailama166116.html.

Chapter 11

1. H. Brown, "The *Other* Brain Also Deals with Many Woes," *International New York Times*, August 23, 2005, http://www.nytimes.com/2005/08/23/health/23gut.html?pagewanted=all&_r=0.

2. "The Mysteries of the Heart," HeartMath, accessed January 4, 2014, http://www.heartmath.org/templates/ihm/articles/infographic/2013/mysteries-of-the-heart/index.php.

3. A. Hadhazy, "Think Twice: How the Gut's 'Second Brain' Influences Mood and Well-Being," *Scientific American*, February 12, 2010.

4. "Intuitive Policing: Emotional/Rational Decision Making in Law Enforcement," *FBI Law Enforcement Bulletin*, February 2004, 1, http://www.au.af.mil/au/awc/awcgate/fbi/intuitive.pdf.

5. P. Gray, "Why Children Protest Going to School: More Evo. Mismatch," *Psychology Today*, November 10, 2011, http://www.psychologytoday.com/blog/freedom-learn/201111/why-children-protest-going-school-more-evo-mismatch.

ACKNOWLEDGMENTS

· · · · · · · · · · · ·

I have been guided towards *The Dolphin Way* my whole life and thus I have a lifetime of people to thank. I cannot name them all individually, but I can name them all collectively—my teachers. My teachers have come in all forms: my loving husband, my devoted parents, my inspiring siblings, my encouraging friends, my supportive colleagues, my reassuring mentors, and my humbling children. It is amazing how much we can learn from others when we are open to receiving what they can offer us.

As a first time author, there are a few people who have fear-lessly guided me into this terrifying place of publishing. I am in deep gratitude to Nick Garrison, my Canadian editor, for bringing his mastery of the art and science of writing to this book and being my "favorite teacher"; Sara Carder, my US editor, for her unwavering optimism for this book's message and her discerning eye for its equally important package; and Arielle Eckstut and David Henry Sterry, my literary "guardian angels" who appeared at just the right time! I would like to thank Armin Brott and Susanna Margolis for their efforts in the early stages of writing and to Claudia Forgas and Mary Ann Blair for finishing the book with precision and care. I am indebted to my courageous agent, Jim Levine, for opening the door and guiding me through it with wisdom, clarity, and kindness. To Ashley Audrain, Trish Bunnett, Charidy Johnston, Vesna Micic, Elizabeth Fischer, and Brianna Yashamita for patiently teaching me the world of publicity, sales, and marketing—thank you all for your boundless energy and enthusiasm. To Scott Loomer and Beth Lockley for working behind the scenes and ensuring I knew Penguin was the right place for me at our fateful first meeting. Thank you to all the talented staff of Levine Greenberg Literary Agency (New York), Penguin Canada (Toronto), Penguin Tarcher (New York), and Shelton Interactive (Austin) for all their hard work and commitment—what amazing teamwork! I am so thankful for Sajan Gill, my bright and innovative research assistant and go-to guy for all that is *The Dolphin Way*.

More than anything, I am truly grateful for the help, dedication, and collaboration of my own personal pod, who encouraged me to start this journey and helped me swim when I was sinking (which was not infrequent)! Simply put, their energy, unconditional support, and love carried me through these last few years.

I must acknowledge that this book does not belong to me alone. Its words also belong to the countless others who have brought them out in me. Its science also belongs to brilliant researchers who have uncovered life's truths. And the essence of this book—its message, its promise, and its spirit—belongs only to Mother Nature, who has gifted us with internal wisdom and limitless joy.

INDEX

. . . .

If you enjoyed this book, visit

www.tarcherbooks.com

and sign up for Tarcher's e-newsletter to receive
special offers, giveaway promotions, and
information on hot upcoming releases.

TARCHER
PENGUIN

Great Lives Begin with Great Ideas

Connect with the Tarcher Community

• • •

Stay in touch with favorite authors!
Enter weekly contests!
Read exclusive excerpts!
Voice your opinions!

Follow us

 Tarcher Books

 @TarcherBooks

If you would like to place a bulk order
of this book, call 1-800-847-5515.